overcoming health anxiety

letting go of your fear of illness

Katherine M. B. Owens, PhD

Martin M. Antony, PhD

New Harbinger Publications, Inc.

Publisher's Note

This publication is designed to provide accurate and authoritative information in regard to the subject matter covered. It is sold with the understanding that the publisher is not engaged in rendering psychological, financial, legal, or other professional services. If expert assistance or counseling is needed, the services of a competent professional should be sought.

Distributed in Canada by Raincoast Books

Copyright © 2011 by Katherine M. B. Owens and Martin M. Antony
New Harbinger Publications, Inc.
5674 Shattuck Avenue
Oakland, CA 94609
www.newharbinger.com

Cover design by Amy Shoup
Text design by Michele Waters-Kermes
Acquired by Catharine Meyers
Edited by Nelda Street

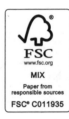

FSC
www.fsc.org
MIX
Paper from
responsible sources
FSC® C011935

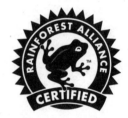

Library of Congress Cataloging in Publication Data

Owens, Katherine M. B.
  Overcoming health anxiety : letting go of your fear of illness / Katherine M.B. Owens and Martin M. Antony.
     p. cm.
  Includes bibliographical references.
  ISBN 978-1-57224-838-0 (pbk.) -- ISBN 978-1-57224-839-7 (pdf e-book)
  1. Hypochondria--Popular works. I. Antony, Martin M. II. Title.
  RC552.H8O94 2011
  616.85'25--dc22
                                    2011012557

33614082338954

Printed in the United States of America

23   22   21

15   14   13   12   11   10   9   8

For Travis, Eadie, and Victoria. Happy eighteenth birthday, Tori!
—Katherine M. B. Owens

For Cynthia.
—Martin M. Antony

Contents

Acknowledgments

The authors wish to thank the many people who helped this project come together by reading chapters and making useful comments and suggestions. Special thanks to Shahlo Mustafaeva, whose careful proofreading and compiling of references made the task of writing that much easier. Also, we are grateful to the staff at New Harbinger Publications for their support, encouragement, and help from the inception of this work to its completion. Finally, we would like to thank all of our clients, whose rich lives helped us formulate case examples we hope the reader can relate to.

Introduction

If you are anxious about your health, this book was written for you. Perhaps you worry a lot about illness, disease, and death. You may experience very frightening physical symptoms or find yourself asking for reassurance from doctors, family, and friends. You might spend time researching the possible causes of your symptoms, but are left feeling more confused than when you started. You may even avoid doctors altogether for fear of discovering that something is seriously wrong.

Your doctor may have told you that there is no physical explanation for your symptoms, that there is no conclusive diagnosis, or that you worry too much about your health. You may also have heard more than your fair share of clichés and well-intentioned reassurances, such as "Don't worry," "Everything will be all right," "We can't find anything wrong," "Think positively," and "Why are you worried about that?" You may have a difficult-to-diagnose illness, fears about your health in the absence of an illness, or both. Health anxiety may leave you feeling tense, upset, and misunderstood. If any of this sounds familiar, this book was written for you.

The costs of your health anxiety to you may include emotional suffering, strained relationships, missed work, lost friendships, and the financial burden of frequent medical appointments, tests, and medications. Health and happiness are often considered our most valuable assets. Without health (or at least the belief that you are mostly healthy), nothing else seems to matter. No wonder undiagnosed illnesses and health anxiety can be so disabling. In addition to your own suffering, the cost to society is difficult to overstate. It is estimated that 10 to 20 percent of the medical budget in the United States is spent on patients with significant health anxiety, costing the American health care system over $250 *billion* per year (Barsky, Orav, and Bates 2005).

Until the early- to mid-1990s, health anxiety was thought to be very difficult to treat. At that time, researchers and therapists began to study cognitive behavioral therapy (CBT) as a treatment for health anxiety. CBT is a form of psychotherapy that has been found to be very successful for treating anxiety-based problems, such as panic disorder, social anxiety, and phobias—so useful that it is now widely recognized by experts as a first-choice treatment for anxiety (Sturmey and Hersen in press; Swinson et al. 2006).

CBT involves learning to change the thoughts and behaviors that contribute to negative emotions, such as anxiety. Your health anxiety may stem from an undiagnosed illness, a serious condition, or a difficult-to-manage disease. Health anxiety can exist in the context of an actual physical illness or in its absence. Either way, CBT can be a powerful tool to improve your quality of life. As with other anxiety-based problems, researchers were quick to discover that CBT is very effective at helping people with health anxiety (Barsky and Ahern 2004). As such, the majority of this book focuses on cognitive and behavioral strategies, with an emphasis on overcoming exaggerated or excessive levels of health anxiety. In addition to CBT, we discuss evidence-based medication treatments and various other approaches that may be helpful, based on preliminary evidence supporting them for other anxiety-related problems. These other strategies include methods for enhancing motivation and learning to tolerate and accept uncomfortable feelings and experiences.

Although there is little research on the use of self-help treatments for health anxiety, there is evidence that CBT-based self-help treatments can be effective for a wide range of anxiety-based problems (Walker, Vincent, and Furer 2009). The strategies described in this book are similar to those that have been found to be useful in studies on the treatment of health anxiety, though these studies have primarily focused on the use of these strategies in the context of therapy with a professional. Whether you decide to work through these strategies on your own or with a therapist, the more you put into the treatment, the more you will get out of it! Unquestionably, the time and effort you devote over the next two to three months will determine how you feel at the end.

We suggest skimming the entire book initially to get a sense of what topics are covered, and then returning to the beginning of the book and reading the chapters more closely in sequential order. The chapters and exercises have been put in this order for a reason. For example, the material on setting goals appears early in the book (you can't really work toward making changes without knowing what changes you want to make). Similarly, information on how to change anxiety-related behaviors comes after learning why making such changes is important.

There will be many different exercises for you to complete as you work through each chapter. Some are short, but some you will have to work through over the course of many weeks. The first step toward overcoming health anxiety is committing to trying the exercises. Although reading and understanding the material is vital, change *will not happen* without your active engagement. We would hate for you to miss out on a better future because we didn't emphasize how important the homework piece of this program is. Get a notebook or journal to use along with this book. Use it to keep track of important points, observations, and tips for yourself, and to complete the exercises that follow. Your notebook or journal should be one that you don't mind carrying around with you.

In general, try to budget one to two weeks for each chapter. This will give you time to read the material and work through the exercises. However, note that some chapters will not take that much time to work through, and others include exercises to practice on an ongoing basis— much longer than just a week or two—as you continue to work through the material in subsequent chapters. As you progress through the book, you will likely find yourself having to put in more time; each section builds on the last, and you will add new exercises on top of ones you've already mastered. Budget for about an hour each day. Although this sounds like a lot of time, health anxiety has already been stealing your time. Whether or not you are dealing with an actual physical illness on top of your anxiety, it is likely that anxious thoughts and behaviors have become time consuming, maladaptive, repetitive, and unproductive.

You may have days when you tell yourself you can take a bit of a break: *Who would know?* Or perhaps you think in absolutes; for example, *If I don't have an hour to spend, why do anything at all?* Or you may think that if you missed a few days or weeks, then all would be lost. Working on your health anxiety may actually increase anxiety in the short term. You wouldn't be the only person who had difficulty planning to do something challenging and perhaps anxiety provoking. If you find that the strategies lead you to have more anxiety early on or you are having difficulty sticking with it, refer to chapter 2 to remind yourself of why it's important to work on your health anxiety now. Asking for support from a close friend or family member may also be helpful.

So, what will be the payoff for all your effort? That's a great question, but only you can answer it! What will you do when your worries about health no longer take up your time and energy (both physical and mental) the way they do now?

chapter 1

Understanding Health Anxiety

If you have health anxiety, you probably worry about your health, focus on bodily symptoms that frighten you, check repeatedly for signs and symptoms related to your health concerns, focus on death or dying, or frequently try to obtain reassurance from family, friends, or doctors. That said, health anxiety means something different for each person. In fact, all readers of this book will understand and experience health anxiety in their own ways. In this chapter you will learn more about the symptoms, causes of, and treatment for health anxiety.

What Is Health Anxiety?

Many of us are irritated with small doubts or questions about our health from time to time. Almost everyone has wondered at some time whether a cough that just won't go away might be something serious, or whether the fellow who sneezed at the next table is contagious. Many people may avoid touching questionable surfaces if they are at a walk-in clinic or hospital, and may wash their hands extra well "just in case." The majority of us are also guilty of occasional online searching to see what our symptoms might mean.

A little anxiety about your physical or mental health can be a very good thing; without it you might never go for a checkup, get a cavity filled, go on vacation, or watch your diet. Not all health anxiety is unrealistic or exaggerated. A twisted ankle that might be broken should be x-rayed, and a sore tooth and swollen face should be checked out by a dentist. Your physician will confirm, for example, that yearly checkups are not unreasonable. On the other hand, excessive health anxiety comes with persistent, unrealistic, maladaptive worries and all the problems that accompany them. In this book we focus mostly on this type of disruptive anxiety. People with moderate or high levels of health anxiety may experience some, or all, of the following:

- Fleeting worries about numerous feelings and sensations (for example, headache, stomach upset, itching, dizziness). These may change from day to day depending on what seems most immediate or important.

- Significant and lasting distress about a few specific feelings and sensations (for example, if your father suffered a serious heart attack at your age, cardiac symptoms might be the only ones that worry you).

- Extreme worry about the possibility of contracting a specific disease (such as cancer, HIV, or multiple sclerosis). This concern might persist or creep back after you have undergone tests and been reasonably reassured by your doctor.

- Fear of public places or situations where you might be exposed to disease or germs (for example, a full airplane, a hospital, or a funeral) because of the anxiety that they could make you seriously ill.

- Anxiety sometimes so strong that you may begin to act in ways that, logically, you know don't make sense. Examples might include avoiding television shows about illness or avoiding reading the obituaries. While on the one hand, it seems obvious that you can't become sick from reading an obituary, on the other hand, doing so can provoke anxiety and discomfort.

Exercise: Identifying the Effects of Health Anxiety

Are there other ways that your health anxiety affects you? If so, record them in your journal, along with any items from the preceding list that apply to you.

Are You A Hypochondriac?

When discussing health anxiety, researchers and clinicians often refer to *hypochondriasis* (a *hypochondriac* is someone who suffers from hypochondriasis). Although hypochondriasis and health anxiety are related, they are not the same thing. Health anxiety is much broader, and can be a feature of depression, various anxiety disorders, chronic illness, pain, and many other problems. Hypochondriasis, on the other hand, is a psychiatric term referring to one particular psychological disorder with very specific diagnostic criteria (American Psychiatric Association 2000). A diagnosis of hypochondriasis requires the following features to be present:

- The person must be preoccupied with a fear of having a serious disease based on misinterpreting the meaning of the physical symptoms.

- The fear has to continue despite medical tests showing that nothing is wrong and despite reassurance from doctors.

- The person is aware on some level that this fear may not be 100 percent accurate.

- ▣ The fear cannot be focused exclusively on a concern about the person's physical appearance.

- ▣ The health-anxiety problems have to be present for at least six months.

Note that several psychiatric conditions involve the *intentional* production of either physical or psychological symptoms. The motivation for this behavior may be to receive attention and care, avoid responsibilities, or get external rewards, such as an insurance settlement or disability pay. We mention this here because this is what people sometimes *mistakenly* believe hypochondriasis means. Hypochondriasis does not involve the intentional production of symptoms, and people with hypochondriasis are not faking their symptoms. Rather, the symptoms are very real, but they misinterpret the symptoms as a sign of serious disease.

Some labels, especially certain psychiatric labels, can be very value laden. This is the case with the terms "hypochondriasis" and "hypochondriac." Over time, the slang use of these terms has become very negative, not to mention inaccurate. In fact, calling someone a hypochondriac may imply that the person is faking the symptoms or is somehow weak. Some might assume that the person's suffering is not justified, or that what the person is experiencing can be overcome simply by trying harder or ignoring the fears. Such assumptions are inaccurate and unfair.

Understanding Anxiety

Anxiety is a common human experience. Whether you are experiencing apprehension about your health, about the big meeting on Monday, or about getting the house in shape before your in-laws arrive in twenty minutes, the experience of anxiety has a surprising sameness. To work on health anxiety, you will need an understanding of anxiety in general.

The Components of Anxiety

Any emotion, including anxiety (about health, public speaking, or your retirement savings), can be broken down into three related elements:

physical sensations, thoughts, and behaviors (Beck and Emery 1985). In this section, we discuss each of these components.

Physical Sensations

We have all experienced the physical sensations that go along with anxiety. If you have sat waiting for a job interview or some important news, you will remember the feeling. You may have experienced a pounding heart, sweaty hands, dry mouth, clumsiness, shakiness, or weak legs. Maybe you even had nausea, blurred vision, difficulty breathing, or confusion. Afterward, you may have found yourself feeling headachy and tired.

The sensations that go along with anxiety are also present when we experience fear or anger; they are there when our adrenaline pumps or we are very excited. For example, imagine how your body might feel as you match up the winning lottery numbers with your lottery ticket! We can even produce these physiological reactions quite easily with stimulants, for example, when we drink too much coffee. Sometimes, these physical sensations come on for no obvious reason. Your brain takes those physical sensations and applies a label to them. What label your brain chooses will depend heavily on the situation. If you've just won the lottery, *Fantastic!* might be a logical attribution. If you are at a horror film, *Scary!* would make more sense. For people who are experiencing anxiety about their health, having these physical symptoms can be frightening, even if they are triggered by some other emotional state.

Anxiety can actually make your symptoms worse. Imagine that you feel anxious about your health, and think that something might *really* be wrong and that your doctor isn't going to catch it before it's too late. These thoughts would worry just about anyone! As you start to worry more, you begin to experience many anxiety sensations. Perhaps your heart pounds, your head pounds, and your stomach turns. Then—and this is the place where people with excessive health anxiety differ from those without it—your mind may incorrectly label the sensations themselves as threatening: *Something's wrong!* But in reality those sensations are simply physical rumblings, no more dangerous than hunger, an itch, or stiffness. When someone is prone to worry about her health, a pounding headache may bring to mind scary stories and worries. Though these disturbances vary from person to person, they might include thoughts about tumors, aneurysms, or meningitis, for example. Suddenly, those meaningless sensations become the focus of extra attention, and the more attention we pay to them, the stronger they feel and the more often they crop up.

Exercise: Your Physical Sensations

Following is a list of physical sensations that most people experience occasionally. Many of these sensations may accompany anxiety or trigger it in people who are anxious about their health. For each sensation in the list, check off whether you experience this sensation on a regular basis (for any reason), and indicate how anxious or frightened you are of experiencing this sensation. Use the following scale for your ratings:

   0 = no anxiety or fear
   1 = mild anxiety or fear
   2 = moderate anxiety or fear
   3 = severe anxiety or fear
   4 = very severe anxiety or fear

Sensation	Check (✓) if you experience on a regular basis	Anxiety (0–4) over experiencing the sensation
Being bothered by bright lights or loud sounds		
Blurry, itchy, or watery eyes		
Breathlessness, difficulty breathing		
Bumps, pimples, whiteheads, blackheads, or ingrown hairs		
Changes in appetite		
Changes in sex drive		
Changes in weight		
Chest pains or tightness		
Chills		

Choking or smothering sensation		
Confusion		
Constipation, fullness, or bloating		
Coughing		
Depersonalization (feeling separate from your body)		
Derealization (things around you seem strange or unreal)		
Difficulty catching your breath		
Difficulty swallowing		
Dizziness		
Dry mouth		
Fatigue or exhaustion		
Feeling hot or cold		
Headache		
Heartburn		
Hot flashes		
Hot, burning, or red face		
Hyperventilation (breathing too quickly and/or too deeply)		
Insomnia		
Itching or burning skin		
Joint tenderness or pain		
"Lump" in your throat		
Lumps under the skin, especially if you rub or touch them		
Muscle pain or cramps		
Muscle stiffness		
Muscles, tendons, or bones "creaking" or "crackling"		
Muscular weakness		
Nasal congestion or "runny" nose		

Nausea or vomiting		
Nightmares		
Poor memory		
Racing or pounding heart, palpitations		
Racing thoughts		
Rashes		
Red eyes		
Ringing ears or distorted hearing		
Rumbling stomach		
Scratchy throat		
Shaking or trembling		
Skin redness		
Skin sensitivity		
Sweating		
Tingling, numbness, "pins and needles"		
Trouble paying attention		
Twitches or tics		
Upset stomach, stomach cramps, or diarrhea		
Other: _____		
Other: _____		
Other: _____		

People with health anxiety focus on specific sensations. These sensations may be symptoms of anxiety, like a rapid heartbeat, a tight throat, or blurred vision, or they may be other garden-variety sensations, such as having digestive problems, experiencing a memory lapse, or noticing lumps and bumps or changes in breathing. There are hundreds of everyday sensations that come and go without harm, including itches, pains, pangs, fatigue, and so on. These sensations are pretty common to the human condition. Such physiological responses are typically not harmful, and usually stem from a benign source, like the caffeine in that cup of tea an hour ago, normal physical processes, or a sleepless night. We also know that worrying (whether about health or a baby shower you're planning) will bring on anxious feelings. In fact, just paying attention to physical sensations can make them more intense. The person with health anxiety often labels these sensations—both normal and anxiety related—as meaningful or dangerous (Taylor and Asmundson 2004). This is called a *misattribution*. We will return in a moment to the ways in which beliefs about sensations and paying attention to sensations can contribute to anxiety.

You may be surprised to learn that throughout this book, we won't try to banish, reduce, or otherwise change these sensations. That's right! Remember, the sensations themselves are not harmful. Really, they are normal. The suffering that you live with and that this book is written to help manage is due to thoughts, beliefs, acts, and emotions, such as fear, avoidance, hopelessness, frustration, and sadness. It is your response to these sensations that we will help you to change, not the sensations themselves.

Thoughts and Attention

Our thoughts play an important role in health anxiety. Excessive anxiety occurs when we interpret a situation as being more dangerous than it actually is. Examples of negative thoughts that may trigger health anxiety include:

- *A sore on my skin means I have skin cancer.*

- *A headache is a sign of a brain tumor.*

- *Having shaky hands means I'm coming down with Parkinson's disease.*

- *A racing heart means I'm having a heart attack.*

- *If my daughter is crying, it means she's seriously ill.*

We will not go into too much detail about the role of thoughts here. Chapter 3 includes a more comprehensive discussion of how thoughts can contribute to health anxiety, as well as exercises designed to help you notice, record, and change these thoughts.

Exercise: Beliefs That Contribute to Your Health Anxiety

In your journal, record some examples of anxiety-provoking beliefs, interpretations, and predictions that run through your mind when you notice sensations or physical feelings that frighten you.

Have you ever had the experience of buying what you thought was an unusual car, only to find afterward that you encountered your car everywhere you looked: in television shows, commercials, magazines, and parking lots and on the road (you can substitute "item of clothing" if you don't have a car)? What you thought was an unusual item turned out to be very common. How is it that you hadn't noticed this before? Once you were mentally "on alert," you noticed things you had never noticed before. You began to see your car (or article of clothing) everywhere because you were looking for it.

Exercise: Attention Experiment

After you read this sentence, close your eyes and focus your attention on how your feet feel for about one minute. Try this now and then come back to the book.

Okay, welcome back. What did you notice? With your mental spotlight pointed at your feet, you probably noticed the pressure where they met the floor, may have sensed what the inside of your shoes or socks felt like, and may have felt your toes touching each other. What words might you use to describe all the sensations you experienced in your feet? Were your feet squashed, relaxed, warm, cold, tingly, sore, itchy?

The most important point to take away from this exercise is the knowledge that these sensations were there all along; you just weren't paying attention. Later, after your attention has moved on to something else (whether it be helping your children with their homework or watching the news), these sensations will continue on with countless others, unnoticed.

As discussed previously, anxiety-provoking thoughts, beliefs, and predictions often determine whether we are likely to experience anxiety in any given situation. Like these thoughts, attention can contribute to anxiety. The more we pay attention to objects, situations, or experiences that make us anxious, the more likely we are to keep the anxiety alive. Just as how noticing someone else yawn can trigger an urge for you to yawn, noticing your anxiety symptoms can affect whether they actually occur.

In early 2009, there was a media frenzy surrounding the H1N1 virus, also known as "swine flu." Before that, there were media reports of E. coli, Listeria, Salmonella, West Nile virus, SARS, "bird flu," and "mad cow" disease, to name a few. During these reports, many people (especially those who are anxious about their health) suddenly noticed every one of their coughs and sneezes. People who are particularly concerned about their well-being notice and pay attention to health information far more than those who are relatively unconcerned. For them—and perhaps you or someone you know—news stories, Web pages, e-mail advertisements, and water-cooler conversations stand out much more when they focus on illness or health-related material. These cues may make you worry about the future, with thoughts such as *What if I catch the flu? What if I get sick and can't work? What if I die? Who will look after the kids?* This is another way in which people with high health anxiety tend to differ from those who don't worry much about their health.

Behaviors

Earlier, we mentioned that behaviors—what you do or don't do—can cause more suffering for people with health anxiety than do the actual physical sensations. Our thoughts are responsible for the connection between our sensations and behaviors. Consider the following examples of situations in which you would experience uncomfortable physical sensations:

- Stubbing your toe really hard as you run to catch the phone

- Feeling nauseous and headachy the morning after overindulging in alcohol

- Feeling bloated and unwell after taking a third helping of food at Thanksgiving even though you were already stuffed

- Feeling an intense, shooting head pain after eating ice cream too quickly

Take a moment and think of what you normally do in each of these situations. If you are like most others, you don't really do much. You may take a second to rub the area, take an aspirin, or slow down on the ice cream; then you would likely turn your attention to other matters. When people without health anxiety notice symptoms or sensations that arise without an obvious source, they don't typically behave differently than they would in the previous examples. They quickly rub the sore foot, complain about the headache, or put a bit of lotion on the rash, and then continue on.

In contrast, people with more health anxiety tend to behave differently when they experience unexplained sensations. If a headache (sensation) develops, for example, without a logical or obvious explanation, the sufferer can make a misattribution of danger: *This headache could be a sign of meningitis* (thought). Many behaviors that are prompted by health anxiety flow *very logically* from such frightening thoughts. Note, we did not say that the behavior, like rushing to the medical clinic, is a logical response to a normal discomfort. The behavior of rushing to the medical clinic is a logical response to the threatening thought *I may have meningitis*. In this case, the thought was mistaken, so the behavior was as well. There are many types of behaviors common to health anxiety, such as checking, investigating, seeking reassurance, avoiding, distracting, exercising to extreme, and overusing vitamins. These behaviors are often referred to as "safety behaviors," because they are designed to protect the person from possible harm. They make perfect sense, given the mistaken thoughts or beliefs behind them. However, in the long run they are not helpful, an issue we will return to in chapter 4.

Exercise: Behaviors That Contribute to Your Health Anxiety

In your journal, record some examples of the things you do when you experience health anxiety, particularly the things you do to reduce your anxiety or to protect yourself from possible danger. These activities may include avoiding situations, seeking reassurance, and engaging in some of the safety behaviors discussed earlier.

Avoiding Emotions

Virtually all cognitive behavioral models of anxiety, including health anxiety, emphasize the roles of sensations, thoughts, and behaviors in establishing and maintaining the cycle of anxiety (and other emotions). If you are like most people, you don't usually enjoy strong negative emotions like fear, anger, frustration, hopelessness, helplessness, worry, angst, disgust, terror, grief, or hate. Depending on life circumstances, most people occasionally find themselves in situations (for example, waiting for a child who was supposed to be home an hour earlier) or thinking thoughts (such as *If my investments keep losing money at this rate, I'll never be able to retire*) that may lead to uncomfortable emotions. At times it can be very tempting to avoid situations or thoughts that lead to such feelings. Think of how many people have stayed in a job they hate in order to avoid the stress of applying and interviewing for a new one.

If you're an anxious person, you are even more likely to avoid. The reasoning goes something like this: if you never let your children out of your sight (for example, by walking them to and from school every day, and prohibiting solo trips to the mall and birthday parties), you might avoid the anxiety that comes from worrying about accidents and kidnappers. You probably know some parents who tend to be this way, albeit likely not to such an extreme. Are these parents less anxious, less worried than most? No? Strangely, all that effort directed at avoiding fear has the opposite effect.

How about people who avoid social gatherings because they worry that they will embarrass themselves? Are these folks extra relaxed and self-satisfied? No, again. Avoiding feelings, including fear, worry, and anxiety about our health, is not helpful. As long as you try to avoid feeling anxious, you will never learn that you can handle the situation and, if necessary, live through the anxiety. In chapter 6, we will review some strategies for dealing with stress.

Putting It All Together: Sensations, Thoughts, Behaviors, and Emotions

Health-related fears vary from person to person. Consider Eleanor, who found herself becoming more and more careful about her health since having her first child four years ago. At first she was simply attentive, washing her hands carefully, eating well, and exercising. As time went by, these steps were not enough to stem the thought *My health is failing*, and the fear and sense of responsibility that came with it. Eleanor's behaviors became more extreme. Every piece of news about illness seemed to apply directly to her. Many of the sensations she experienced—fatigue, weight loss, dry skin, rapid pulse, insomnia—fit the descriptions of serious diseases. She found herself going to the doctor every few weeks to check on one symptom or another.

After these appointments Eleanor felt better for a short while, but her anxiety quickly returned, along with nagging doubts about whether the doctor might have missed something, whether she had reported all her symptoms correctly, or whether she might have misunderstood the results. She felt trapped and hopeless as the cycle started again. Most recently, Eleanor was unable to visit her mother in the hospital; the likelihood of catching an infection just felt too great to take the risk. If Eleanor caught a debilitating illness, who would take care of her kids? She felt sick just thinking about it, but the guilt remained.

Let's identify some of the facets of Eleanor's health anxiety. Her story might be similar to yours or quite different. Take a moment to read over Eleanor's experiences again. Try to identify some of her sensations, thoughts, behaviors, and emotions.

Here are some examples you might have identified after a second reading.

Sensations	Thoughts	Behaviors	Emotions
Fatigue	My health is failing.	Washing	Afraid
Weight loss	My symptoms suggest a terrible illness.	Diet	Anxious
Dry skin	The doctor missed something this time.	Exercise	Responsible
Insomnia	The doctor didn't understand what I was trying to say.	Read health news	Trapped
Rapid pulse	What if I'm remembering wrong?	Go to doctor	Hopeless
Sick feeling	Hospitals are covered with germs.	Avoid hospital	Guilty
	The risk of catching an infection at the hospital is high.		
	I could become really sick or even die.		
	Who will care for the kids?		

Health Anxiety in the Context of Actual Physical Illness

It is sometimes assumed that only those without illness or disease can be considered to have health anxiety. After all, excessive concern is part of the definition, and those with demonstrable illnesses have reason enough to worry, right? Not necessarily. Anyone can demonstrate fear, anxiety, or worry that is greater than might be expected in the given situation, or is of a severity that is bothersome or interferes with important aspects of the person's life, including relationships, work, or school.

Health anxiety is seen in people with a wide variety of general medical conditions, such as cancer, multiple sclerosis, diabetes, allergies, and high blood pressure (see, for example, Furer, Walker, and Stein 2007).

Consider Eduardo, a driven, hardworking, and highly successful businessman. He put in long hours, worked evenings and weekends, and spent many hours entertaining clients in fancy restaurants and trendy bars. His personality fit the label commonly referred to as "type A." During a routine checkup, Eduardo's doctor told him he needed to slow down and take his health more seriously, because he had mild coronary heart disease. Eduardo became terrified that he would keel over from a heart attack at any moment. All his wealth and power would mean nothing because he would be dead.

Eduardo began to give up staying in touch with his business contacts. Some days he could not bear to stay in the office for more than a few minutes, and quickly drove home to lie down, with his heart pounding in fear. Eduardo stopped sharing in the family meals, feeling it was better for his digestion if he ate bland items in quiet solitude. He quit drinking coffee, tea, and soda, because he experienced frightening sensations from the caffeine. Whenever he noticed his heart beating quickly, Eduardo sat down. He also started to avoid saunas, sex, and exercise, for fear of the sensations they produced. Eduardo's life was becoming less and less enjoyable, and his world shrank by the day.

Eduardo's story provides an example of how exaggerated health anxiety can be present even in a person with a demonstrated medical concern. The information in this book may be helpful regardless of whether you have an actual medical complaint or disease.

Health Anxiety in the Context of Another Psychological Disorder

People with moderate or severe health anxiety are more likely to experience other psychological problems (for example, other anxiety disorders, depression, or alcohol or drug abuse) than people who don't have excessive anxiety about their health. These other conditions often involve an element of health anxiety. Essentially, your health anxiety may stand on its own or be a facet of another disorder. Three conditions are particularly common among people with high health anxiety: generalized anxiety disorder, depression, and panic disorder. We mention them here because if one of these conditions is a prominent issue for you, you may need to work on it before you will feel a significant decrease in your health anxiety. By analogy, if your scratchy throat stands on its own, a lozenge will likely help; if your scratchy throat stems from a cat allergy, a lozenge might help, but removing yourself from an environment with cat dander should be your first consideration.

Generalized anxiety disorder can be distinguished from uncomplicated health anxiety, in part, by the wide variety of worries present—far more than someone else in your same position might experience. People with generalized anxiety disorder often worry about their health, but they also worry about their families, personal safety, work, school, money, and various other topics. They experience their worries as difficult to control and leading to irritability, difficulty sleeping, and other associated symptoms. Depression can also be differentiated from health anxiety by: sadness, loss of interest, appetite changes, sleep changes, feelings of agitation or slowing down, fatigue, feelings of worthlessness or excessive guilt, poor concentration, or thoughts of death or suicide. Finally, people with panic disorder experience rushes of panic that occur out of the blue (without any obvious trigger or cause), and that are associated with a variety of uncomfortable and frightening sensations. They often worry about the health-related consequences of their panic attacks (for example, that they may die, faint, or have a heart attack). If you experience recurrent, unexpected panic attacks, treatment for panic disorder may be an important step in learning to handle your health fears.

The information in this book will likely be useful regardless of whether you experience some of these other problems in addition to your health anxiety. However, when deciding which problem to treat first, it may be helpful to think about which problem is affecting your life the most at this time. For example, if you experience depression that is much more severe than your health anxiety, we recommend that you seek treatment for your depression before trying to tackle your health anxiety. Your family physician or a mental health professional (a psychologist or psychiatrist, for example) can help you to figure out what sorts of problems you are experiencing in addition to your health anxiety, and which problems should be treated first.

What Causes Health Anxiety?

Many factors influence the ways in which people differ. For example, your weight may depend on genetics, the influence of the media (for example, advertising), the attitudes of those around you, the availability of different foods, your experiences, stress level, personal tastes, and health. The same is true for health anxiety. Psychological variations are thought to be determined, in part, by biological factors (for example, genetics) and also by psychological factors (such as life experiences).

A genetic vulnerability to developing health anxiety does not mean that you are ordained from birth to become anxious about illness and disease but, rather, that you are more likely to be anxious than someone who doesn't have this vulnerability. By way of analogy, consider the tendency to get sunburned. We all know that people who are very fair can easily find themselves nursing a sunburn. Now, if they are careful, have a preference for long-sleeved shirts and hats, or live where it's often overcast, these people may never experience a sunburn; they are just more likely than others to burn, given certain environmental factors.

The Role of Genetics

It will probably come as no surprise to hear that you are more likely to experience health anxiety if your immediate relatives (for example, your parents or siblings) also experience excessive health anxiety. Of course, knowing that health anxiety runs in families does not mean that the transmission of health anxiety from one generation to the next is solely, or even mostly, genetic. Although we inherit our genetic makeup from our parents, our personalities are also influenced by what we learn from our parents. Studies of twins (Taylor et al. 2006) show that some features of health anxiety are moderately heritable; that is, they are influenced by both genetic and environmental factors.

The Role of Social and Cultural Factors

From a social perspective, there are many experiences, institutions, and beliefs that you probably share with others in the wider culture in which you live, any of which can influence your tendency to be anxious about your health.

The Role of the Media in Health Anxiety

One sociocultural institution that you share with those around you is the media: books, movies, newspapers, magazines, television (fictional shows, news stories, advertisements, and reality television), and the Internet. As technology becomes more advanced, the media gives us access to an overwhelming and real-time deluge of health information (and misinformation).

On any given day, we can find news stories about illness, disease, viruses, bacteria, and death. Many news websites have entire sections dedicated to illness (though ironically, they tend to call these "Health" sections). These Web pages are filled with information about contagious and infectious diseases and every sort of illness imaginable, and they encourage worry where it is not needed. This sort of information invariably increases health anxiety. Thinking about this logically, you have to wonder if the world is really more rife with illness than it was seventy-five or a hundred years ago! Of course not; humans are actually healthier now and live longer than ever before.

Another problem with relying on the media for information about health and disease is that good news is boring. Not only are we inundated with far more information than we need, what is reported and written about has a definite negative slant. We never hear about the billions of people who do not contract H1N1, Salmonella, or flesh-eating bacteria, for example. When incidents of medical error or misdiagnosis happen, they are quickly transmitted across the globe. We hear stories of travelers returning home with mysterious illnesses, labs mixing up results, and doctors prescribing medications in error. What we do not hear about are the numerous times that everything goes right for every one mistake. It makes perfect sense that we might believe that illness and disease are around every corner. That's what we read in the paper, see online, and watch on the news.

A final problem with relying on the media for health information is their tendency to report *relative* risks rather than *absolute* risks. It is not uncommon to see headlines that say "People who eat X are five times more likely to develop heart disease" or "People who do Y are three times as likely to develop cancer." Without knowing the actual numbers, these sorts of statements are almost meaningless. For example, if the odds of developing a particular disease are one in one hundred thousand, and eating a particular food multiplies that risk by five, that would bring the risk of developing the illness to one in twenty thousand, still very low! On the other hand, if the risk is initially one in five, and eating a particular food multiplies the risk by five, then your risk increases to 100 percent, very high! So, without knowing the actual rate of a disease, knowing that some variable increases or decreases the risk by a factor of five tells you nothing about your likelihood of developing the illness. Television news, magazines, and newspapers rarely report absolute numbers when they discuss risk factors for particular diseases. Instead they often just report the amount by which the risk increases or decreases, given some factor of interest (such as diet, exercise, stress, age, smoking, and so on).

Your Individual Environment

You share more with your relatives than just genetics and media influences. Shared environmental factors may contribute to the transmission of psychological problems from one generation to the next. Though these environmental conditions differ for each family, they may include factors such as race, culture, language, educational attainment, economic and social status, attitudes, traditions, habits, and even attractiveness. Very different experiences while growing up might affect a wide range of beliefs children might hold, including the ways in which they interpret the physical sensations we all experience.

It has been demonstrated that cultural factors influence how people interpret bodily changes and whether they seek medical care. For example, attention to the heart, circulation, and blood pressure is particularly common in Germany; concerns with dizziness or faintness are especially common in certain Caribbean cultures; and immunological or viral symptoms (such as chemical sensitivity, SARS, and "swine flu") are common in the United States and Canada (Escobar et al. 2001). A person from Germany (or who was raised by people with a German heritage) might find a slow heartbeat, "skipped beats," or cold hands very frightening, and a cause for alarm or action, compared to a person raised in the Caribbean or the United States, who might not even notice these sensations.

Clearly, you have learned many rules (both formal and "unwritten") based on the environment in which you live. Some of this learning is purposeful, such as what side of the road to drive on and which vaccinations to have your children get. A great deal of what you know has been absorbed without conscious effort (for example, how to dress for a job interview versus a day at the beach, how long to maintain direct eye contact in a conversation before glancing away or down, or how to politely accept a compliment). Many of these learned beliefs and opinions feel like objective facts. Examples of learned assumptions concerning health include any of these beliefs:

- *Dying should take place in the hospital.*

- *Children should not be allowed to put dirty objects in their mouths.*

- *Body fat is unhealthy.*

- *Those with a fever must stay home from work or school.*

- *Bleeding should always be stopped.*

There are, in fact, many cultures and contexts in which these assumptions are not considered fact. If you hold some of these beliefs, you may be surprised to learn that the people who do not share these beliefs are not less healthy or more anxious as a result.

Exercise: Your Beliefs

Think for a moment about some of your own beliefs about what "healthy" means. What about wellness, illness, disease, and death? Some of your responses will reflect your own personal thoughts, whereas others will mirror what you have learned from those around you. Record your responses in your journal.

Experience with Illness and Death

In addition to broad cultural, social, and environmental factors, our own personal experiences with illness, disability, disease, or death tend to shape how we feel about each of these topics. When events are experienced as inexplicable, frightening, horrific, or shocking, they may be met with a sense of helplessness, hopelessness, futility, or dread, potentially leading to excessive health concerns. Anxiety can be immediate or may develop slowly over time. Experiences that may fall into this category can take place at any time in your life and may include:

- A sudden or unexpected illness in yourself or someone else (for example, years ago a colleague developed bacterial meningitis, and since then, you find yourself frightened and tense whenever you have a headache or sore neck)

- Hearing about a frightening medical experience (for example, you pay particular attention to abdominal sensations and appetite changes after reading a newspaper article describing the case of a woman who was told she had nothing to worry about and then died of pancreatic cancer six weeks later)

- The death of a friend, loved one, or someone to whom you can relate (for example, a healthy brother-in-law dies from a heart attack, after which you find yourself avoiding activities that make your heart pound)

- ▣ A long-term or protracted illness in yourself or someone else (for example, living with a parent with poorly controlled diabetes may heighten your sensitivity to illness in general)

- ▣ A serious or protracted disability in yourself or someone else (for example, after losing partial sight in one eye due to a detached retina you had ignored, you may find yourself going to the emergency room every time your vision is fuzzy or your eyes feel strained)

Learned Anxiety

When an experience changes us, learning takes place. Based on our experiences, we change our thoughts, behaviors, and emotional responses. For example, you may be nervous around loaded guns, but as a baby, you weren't, because you had not learned to fear them yet. Other adults who are familiar with weapons (for example, soldiers) must unlearn this fear. All of our health behaviors are learned, from monitoring heart rate to looking up symptoms online to asking for reassurance, visiting the hospital, or repeatedly checking our symptoms. Our responses to most physical sensations are learned as well. When experiencing nausea, for example, some people have learned to ignore it, some take medication, some stop what they are doing and find a spot to rest, and others begin a mental inventory, checking in to see how the rest of the body feels and closely monitoring the stomach.

Humans (and all animals) learn in a few particular ways:

- ▣ **Reinforcement:** A learning process that *increases* the likelihood of a behavior in the future, reinforcement involves two steps: (1) an action (mental or physical), and (2) a response to that action that makes you more likely to behave the same way again. For example, if you go to work (action) and get a paycheck every two weeks (positive response), you will likely keep going to work. Going back to Eduardo, from earlier in the chapter, as soon as he noticed his heart pounding, he sat down (action). His heart rate eventually returned to normal (positive response). The next time Eduardo felt his heart pounding or racing, he was more likely to stop what he was doing and sit down.

▣ **Punishment:** Punishment is a learning process that *decreases* the likelihood of a behavior in the future. Like reinforcement, it also involves two steps: (1) an action (mental or physical), and (2) a response to that action that makes you less likely to behave the same way again. After a dog pees on the carpet (action) and gets chased into his doghouse by an angry owner waving a newspaper (negative response), the dog will probably be less likely to do the same again. After a strenuous workout (action), Eduardo noticed his heart pounding; because he could see his chest moving with each beat and found this terrifying (negative response), he was sure he had done something to worsen his mild heart disease. Because this was a frightening experience, Eduardo was much less inclined to go back to the gym.

▣ **Observation and information:** You also learn by observing others or by hearing about their experiences. You don't have to be run over to look both ways before crossing the street; being told by your parents about the consequences of crossing the street without looking both ways was probably enough to ensure that you learned the lesson. Likewise, you don't have to experience lung cancer firsthand to know that it's best to avoid smoking.

Exercise: Factors That Have Contributed to Your Anxiety

In your journal, write each of the following headings at the top of a separate blank page:

- Inherited or familial factors

- Cultural factors (including the media)

- Experiences with illness or death

- Learning experiences (reinforcement, punishment, and observation and information)

Take some time to think of examples for each of these factors that may have contributed to the development (and maintenance) of some of your health anxieties. Spend about ten minutes on each page, and write down as many possibilities as you can think of for each. You don't have to do this all at once; for example, you might try a couple today and finish the rest tomorrow. Over the coming weeks, add examples as you think of them.

You will probably find that the sensations, thoughts, and behaviors that accompany your health anxiety did not come out of the blue. In fact there are likely quite a few factors that contributed to your health anxiety and concerns about illness. But that doesn't mean that your health anxiety is necessary, protective, useful, or unchangeable.

In Brief...

At this point you know what health anxiety is, and you have been introduced to the cognitive behavioral method. In chapter 2 you will be invited to explore your motivators and set goals. You are going to envision a better future; after all, why else would you want to change?

chapter 2

Investment in Change

The changes this book is intended to help you achieve may seem out of reach. For now, we ask that you put aside any reservations you have and view this treatment as an experiment designed to test your beliefs about whether this approach will work for you. Throughout this program, you will challenge the thoughts and behaviors that, for all intents and purposes, have seemed to keep you safe thus far. Rather than avoid uncomfortable sensations and emotions, you will go out of your way to experience these feelings until they are no longer scary. To work through these challenges, you must make a commitment to the process of change.

Why Change Often Seems Difficult

Let's face it, if changing the thoughts and behaviors that perpetuate health anxiety were an easy task, if you were completely convinced that there was no risk involved, you would have done it by now! On one hand, it may seem that there are advantages to these anxious thoughts and behaviors. In fact, all human behavior has some benefit. On the other hand, there is no doubt that experiencing health anxiety can be very costly. It may have cost you peace of mind, kept you from enjoying activities, or caused arguments and distress. Perhaps some of the cost has been financial. You may also have felt sad, guilty, or frustrated. Sadly and ironically, some people with severe health anxiety may even think about suicide at times.

For you to have continued checking, researching, looking for reassurance, avoiding medical situations, and so on, the benefits must have seemingly outweighed the costs—at least until now. Consider Jin. Jin had been told by his family doctor that he had mildly elevated blood pressure. At first, he didn't worry about it that much, but over time, his anxiety increased. Jin became acutely aware of his physical sensations. When he was exercising, excited, or nervous, Jin's heart would pound, his face and ears would get blotchy and red, and he would become flushed and sweaty. Jin was completely convinced that these symptoms indicated that his blood pressure was becoming dangerously high and that he was close to having a stroke.

Jin stopped going anywhere that made him anxious or excited, and would immediately stop whatever he was doing if the symptoms came on. He began to miss work and eventually lost his job. Although in dire straits financially, he was far too embarrassed to apply for disability pay or social assistance. His relationship was in shambles, and he certainly didn't want his kids to know what was going on. On one hand, Jin knew that if he didn't make some changes, the life he was living would never improve. On the other hand, he found himself completely unable to behave differently for more than a moment or two.

Many people have found ways to face and conquer difficult challenges, just like Jin's health anxiety. This chapter will help you to evaluate whether you are ready for change and will provide strategies for enhancing your motivation for change. The strategies in this chapter are based, in part, on James Prochaska and Carlo DiClemente's (1983) Stages of Change model, as well as motivational enhancement techniques developed by William Miller and Stephen Rollnick (2002). Both approaches are designed to help people who are trying to make a difficult change, such as overcoming a serious addiction or losing a large amount of weight.

Stages of Change

The Stages of Change model proposes six loosely defined steps that we move through as we try to make a difficult change in our lives (Prochaska and DiClemente 1983). Some people may move through these stages at a nice, even pace, but most people jump forward, inch back, and occasionally move back and forth between the stages. Ambivalence about change (and the effort required) is normal. It is up to you to decide for yourself when you are ready to move forward. This is especially important in the context of this book. Soon we will encourage you to confront your most feared thoughts, situations, sensations, and emotions, and to stop engaging in the safety behaviors (for example, seeking reassurance) you normally use to feel better. There is really no way this can be forced on you; long-term change cannot be externally imposed on you. Rather, you need to be a willing and engaged participant. Once that happens, there will be no limit to your potential success! The six stages of change are as follows.

Precontemplation. At this stage, you have not yet acknowledged, recognized, or accepted that there is a problem. If you bought this book for yourself, you are probably past this stage (though you may remember a time when you were at this stage). If you are reading this book because you believe a loved one has health anxiety, it is possible that your loved one is in this stage.

Contemplation. In this stage, you acknowledge that there is a problem, but might not be willing or able to work on it yet.

Preparation. At this stage, you have made a commitment to change and have taken some small steps toward changing (for example, purchasing this book).

Action. In the action stage, you are actively taking steps to change problematic behaviors, relying on your own motivation and willpower, and purposefully moving toward your goals (for example, reading this book and completing the exercises).

Maintenance. Once you have made a change, maintenance is the process of being vigilant about keeping it up.

Relapse. Relapse is a return to old patterns and behaviors. In the case of overcoming anxiety, most people are able to maintain the gains they have made, for the most part. Nevertheless, some return of anxiety is common, and can happen to the best of us.

Many people experience a return of symptoms that can last anywhere from moments to long periods of time. You may have experienced giving up on an exercise or diet program, or on your attempts to quit smoking, drinking, or chewing your nails. Or, you may sometimes find yourself procrastinating after a nice period of productivity. Oh, and let's not forget about New Year's resolutions! A lapse itself is not failure; it's what you do next that counts. If you notice a return to your old anxious ways of behaving, review the material that you found helpful in the past and get right back into the action stage. In fact, you may read this chapter or section a second time to help you get "back on the wagon," so to speak. If you find yourself reading this material a second (or third or forth) time, you are already back in either the preparation or action stage, and ready to reclaim your positive changes!

Exercise: How Ready Are You for Change?

Now is a good time to get an idea of your current readiness. Take a moment to think about the following questions:

- From what you read in the introduction and chapter 1, does it seem as if health anxiety may be playing some role in your suffering?

- Do you believe (even a bit) that you could learn new techniques that might help you change your thoughts and actions?

- Are you willing to try the strategies described in this book?

- When?

With these thoughts about readiness in mind, decide where you fit, right now, on the following scale. There is no right answer; just put a check mark on the line wherever seems most appropriate, even if it is between two numbers.

1	2	3	4	5	6	7
There is nothing I can or need to change.	Excessive anxiety about my health may be causing me difficulty.	Excessive anxiety about my health is a problem, but I'm not ready to work on it.	I am ready to begin work on my health anxiety in the next few months.	I am ready, now, to change my thoughts and behaviors.	I am making little changes (such as, gathering information about health anxiety).	I am already making real changes in my thoughts and behaviors about my health.

The preceding numbers roughly correlate to the Stages of Change (1 = precontemplation, 3 = contemplation, 5 = preparation, 7 = action).

Exercise: Your Motivations and Perceived Barriers at a Glance

In the next section we will go into a lot more detail about your motivators. For now, start a new page in your journal and try to answer these two questions based on where you marked your readiness on the previous number line.

1. If you made your mark anywhere other than 1, you have some desire or motivation to see things change. Why do you think your check mark wasn't farther to the left, closer to 1? For example, *Why was my mark just shy of 3? I really can't fool myself anymore into thinking this is normal. I have friends with serious illnesses (one of whom is probably dying!) who have a higher quality of life than I do. Physical health alone cannot possibly be the only variable.*

2. If you made your mark anywhere other than 7, you perceive some barriers to full-out change. Why do you think your check mark wasn't farther to the right, closer to 7? For

example, *If I start down this path of examining the role of psychological factors in my health problems, no one will ever take my real health concerns seriously.*

This exercise is important to your personal growth, so be thorough with your answers.

Enhancing Your Motivation

In this section you will consider several strategies for enhancing motivation (Miller and Rollnick 2002). We will walk you through the exercises, but the direction you take will be your own. In a nutshell, the fact that you are reading this book suggests that there is a gap or disconnect between where you are and where you want to be, a gap between your day-to-day experience and what you intrinsically value—your wishes and hopes. If there weren't a gap (in other words, if your life were exactly how you want it to be), there would be no reason to continue with this book. This difference between where you are and where you would like to be is sometimes called *dissonance*. The greater the dissonance (or, the farther your current situation is from where you want or need it to be), the greater your motivation to change! There are two important steps to highlight this dissonance and thereby increase your motivation for change:

1. Increase your awareness of the problems and consequences health anxiety is causing.

2. Develop a detailed picture of a better future.

Jin's life (and the lives of his wife and kids) was miserable, yet he was having difficulty committing to change. Whenever he thought about it, or if anyone suggested trying something new, his mind immediately went into "yes, but" mode. Everyone has "yes, but" moments from time to time. We understand the facts and logic, and yet feel ambivalent about change. The following are some pretty common real-life examples of ambivalence:

▣ *Smoking is dangerous and expensive; I should quit. Yes, but it would cost just as much to go on the patch, I'd gain a bunch of weight if I quit, I work so hard and smoking is my only luxury, and...*

▣ *This job makes me miserable; I should find something better. Yes, but I could never find something else that pays this well; I'm too shy to interview; we might move in the next few years, so there's no point in getting comfortable somewhere new; and...*

▣ *We're falling farther into debt every month, so the family needs to set a budget. Yes, but that would be a lot of work, it would seem too restrictive, there would be so many exceptions that there's no point, and...*

Sound familiar? All of us can be our own worst enemies when it comes to talking ourselves *out* of action. In this next exercise, you will focus on the first half of these statements, minus the "yes, buts!"

Exercise: The Problem with Health Anxiety

The goal of this exercise is to think about the problems health anxiety causes for you and people around you. Examples might include behaviors related to health anxiety, ways of looking at the world, unpleasant emotions, missed work, or negative effects on your relationships. In your journal, list some of the biggest problems that anxiety about your health is causing for you or others in your life. To get started, you might ask yourself the following questions:

▣ *Have my health fears had any negative effect on my mood or mental health?*

▣ *Have I been getting as much pleasure from life as I would like?*

▣ *Are there any life goals that I have given up on or forgotten about as my health concerns have taken center stage?*

▣ *Have I failed, or not done as well as I'd have liked to, in any of my work, school, or home responsibilities because of health fears? Have I missed any work or not given my full effort and attention to things I need to get done?*

▣ *Has health anxiety put a strain on my relationship with my partner? How about with my children, parents, or siblings? In what ways?*

▣ *If I were to ask important others in my life how my health fears and behaviors have affected them, what might they say? (If you aren't sure, go ahead and ask them.)*

▣ *Has health anxiety put a strain on any of my friendships or relationships with coworkers and colleagues?*

▣ *Have my health fears, complaints, and need for reassurance affected my relationship with my physician? Have I ever thought that I might have to switch doctors?*

▣ *Have I had to pay for any medication, tests, or appointments that may not have been completely necessary or useful?*

▣ *Have my finances been affected by my health in any other ways?*

▣ *How much effort do I expend thinking about, monitoring, or researching my health?*

▣ *Do I ever drink alcohol or use drugs (prescription or nonprescription) to cope with anxiety?*

▣ *Some people with health anxiety have a history of medical tests, investigations, and referrals to specialists that fail to turn up a definitive physical disorder. Is this the case for me? If so, is it possible that doctors may be less likely to take my concerns seriously down the road?*

▣ *Are there any important situations I have missed out on because of health worries (for example, a family gathering, visiting a new baby at the hospital)?*

🔲 *Are there simple pleasures I am missing out on (for example, going to a football game, enjoying a hot cup of coffee, watching my favorite medical drama on television)?*

Be as specific as possible. Instead of just writing, "My relationship with the kids is terrible," think about the details. How is it terrible? Perhaps you don't spend enough time with them, you avoid them if they are sick, or you stay away from their school. Maybe your children look at you as if you're crazy when you start talking about your fears, or perhaps they are becoming anxious themselves. This kind of specific information is what you need to record. You may even need a few pages. Remember, the greater the gap between where you are and where you want to be, the more motivation you will find. Don't skip this exercise; you will return to these struggles in the coming weeks. Your sense of investment or your belief that life can be better may tip the scale in favor of change, preparing you for action.

When Jin completed this exercise, he was able to think of many reasons why he wanted to change. Next, you'll find his answers as examples.

Some of the Problems My Health Fears Have Caused:

- *I used to love camping. I'd chop wood while my wife and kids set up the tent. We haven't been able to do that in four years.*

- *My children are learning to be afraid of illness.*

- *I am becoming depressed.*

- *The house is falling apart; I have been letting the repairs and upkeep slide.*

- *I miss putting on a shirt and tie in the morning and heading off to the office. Going to work made me feel that I was doing something worthwhile.*

- *Sipping a cup of hot coffee while I read the paper used to be enjoyable, but now I'm too scared of the symptoms it brings on.*

- *I think my doctor is starting to avoid me; she postponed our last two appointments.*

- *I can't even enjoy sex (which I really liked before) without worrying about my blood pressure.*

- *Despite all these efforts to be healthy and safe, I feel worse and worse.*

- *Our friends don't invite us over anymore. Half the time we would have to cancel because of my anxiety; the rest of the time I made them uncomfortable by constantly talking about disease statistics.*

When you can't think of any more ways in which health anxiety is disrupting your life, ask your partner, family members, or close friends to contribute their impressions and observations. You may be surprised. Jin was shocked to learn that his wife missed cuddling on the sofa while watching their favorite medical drama. He hadn't even realized that this was something they had long since quit doing.

Exercise: A Brighter Future

Now that you have a fairly clear picture of what your health anxiety is costing you, how about the potential for gain? The goal of this exercise is to envision what your life might look and feel like if you no longer had to worry about your health. Start a new page in your journal for this exercise. To get started, you might ponder the following questions:

- If you woke up tomorrow and had no worries or concerns about your health, how would your life look different?

- If your physical sensations (for example, changes in appetite, palpitations, or difficulty breathing) were accounted for completely by a benign or insignificant explanation that didn't worry you in the least, what would this mean for you?

- Why did you decide to open this book and read what you've read so far?

- How would the lives of your family or close friends be different if you no longer acted on your health fears? Are there activities you would do with friends and family that you don't do now?

- How would your work, household responsibilities, or schooling benefit from the extra time and attention you could have?

- If health anxiety has cost you monetarily, what would you rather spend your money on?

- In the last exercise, you listed some simple pleasures you're missing out on. Now list some simple pleasures you would build back into your life if you were suddenly no longer anxious about your health. These might be the same ones you thought about missing earlier, or they might not.

- How might your physical health benefit if you learned to manage your anxiety?

- In the last exercise, you listed some life goals that you have all but given up on or forgotten. If you were able to start working toward some of these goals again, why would that matter? What would be the gains to you and others?

- Take a moment to picture yourself feeling at ease, happy, unfazed, and pleased with your life. What would it mean for you to be able to feel like this more often?

Jin found this exercise more difficult than the one before; he had been anxious about his health so long that he had almost lost sight of what life could be like. With some extra effort (for example, he paid attention to what a normal life might look like by observing others in his life and on television), Jin came up with lots of reasons to make changes. Next, you will find a small sample of his reasons.

What My Life Could Be:

- *I would smile more often at my family and others.*

- *After the kids are in bed, I would watch "House" and snuggle with my wife on the sofa.*

- *When I stopped working, I was making a decent salary. If I could get back into a similar position, we could begin to take family vacations again.*

- *If we didn't have to worry about money, my wife could invite all her relatives over for a big summer barbeque, as we used to do.*

- *My children would grow up feeling more confident and less afraid.*

- *I would be able to have a healthy love life again.*

- *I could volunteer at the hospital, in a seniors' home, or at the animal shelter.*

- *Once I'm less anxious (and back at work), I will have way more self-confidence. In turn, I'll be a better employee, colleague, husband, dad, and friend.*

- *My family doctor would be absolutely thrilled if I could give up some of this worry.*

When you can't think of any more ways in which managing your health anxiety would be beneficial, ask your significant other or one or more close friends or relatives to contribute their impressions and observations. Finally, take a moment to ask yourself *why* each of your points is worth working for. For example, Jin had to think about why a healthy love life was important to him.

Exercise: Now, How Ready Are You for Change?

If it has been a day or two since you worked on the last two exercises, take a moment to read over your responses again. With these thoughts about readiness in mind, decide where you fit, right now, on the following scale. Like last time, there is no right answer; just put a check mark on the line.

1	2	3	4	5	6	7
There is nothing I can or need to change.	Excessive anxiety about my health may be causing me difficulty.	Excessive anxiety about my health is a problem, but I'm not ready to work on it.	I am ready to begin work on my health anxiety in the next few months.	I am ready, now, to change my thoughts and behaviors.	I am making little changes (such as, gathering information about health anxiety).	I am already making real changes in my thoughts and behaviors about my health.

It's Up to You

You may find that your motivation has increased since you began reading this chapter; that is, your readiness to change may have moved closer to 7. The goal of this chapter has been to help you move from thinking about change or taking small steps toward action to feeling ready to actively behave in new ways. If you are reading this because someone else told, asked, or begged you to, you may find yourself moving closer to change, but you may not be quite ready yet. That's all right! You can put this book wherever you'll see it—on the bathroom counter, beside the fridge, or under the TV remote—and come back to it when *you* are ready. Readiness to change has to come from you. Don't get us wrong; we're not saying you can't engage in this, in part, for someone you care about, but the choice to act has to be your own.

Setting Realistic Goals

Now that you feel more invested in change (just look at all the important reasons for change you just came up with), it's time to set some goals. Identifying your goals will help keep you motivated and focused as you work toward change.

Nowhere has goal setting been as well researched and thought out as in the fields of business and management. It is from these fields that we have learned the importance of making your goal specific, measurable, attainable, relevant, and timely, or SMART, which is also known as SMART goal setting (Locke 1968). The SMART method is a simple, yet powerful, way to set goals. In the next sections, we discuss how you can set goals you will be most likely to achieve.

Specific. Make sure the goals you set are very *detailed and clear*. The more detailed your goal, the more likely that you will be able to tell if you are actively working toward it and whether you have achieved it. Take Travis, for example. At first he thought "to feel less anxious" would be a good goal to work toward. When asked to make this goal more specific, he was able to come up with a number of smaller, more specific objectives, such as "to watch the 6:00 p.m. news each day, including stories about illness and disease, while managing my anxiety." Another example of a vague goal that Travis had originally set was "to ignore my heart rate." When he gave it some thought, Travis was able to come up with a much more specific goal: "to take my pulse and blood pressure no more than once a week."

Measurable. Create goals for which you can measure change and outcome. This way you can see your own progress. Being specific goes a long way toward ensuring that a goal is measurable; vague goals are hard to measure. The goal "to feel less anxious" is vague, as mentioned earlier, but it's also difficult to measure. For example, how might Travis know when he was halfway there? On the other hand, the more specific goals Travis identified are also easy to measure. He was able to track his success at watching the news, including segments about illness, each day. He was also able to measure how often he was assessing his blood pressure and pulse. Those around him could easily confirm whether he was doing this more or less than he had committed to.

Attainable. The goals you set for yourself need to be meaningful and important to you. As such, it is reasonable to expect that meeting your goals will be challenging to some extent. On the other hand, if you set goals that are too far out of reach, you probably won't fully commit to them. Although you may start with the best of intentions, goals that are not attainable may prevent you from giving them your best. This is another reason why you need to set your own targets: what seems simple to your significant other may not be so for you. "To stop going to the doctor" was not attainable for Travis and likely would not be attainable or desirable for most people; all of us have to see a physician at some point. "To agree on a schedule of appointments with my doctor, eventually going every six months" was much more reasonable and attainable for Travis. This was the kind of goal he could work toward (note, it's also specific and measurable).

Relevant. To be relevant to you, each of your specific goals around health anxiety should relate to your vision of the future, and to your own personal values. For example, Travis wanted his future to be driven by family relationships; he wanted his wife, kids, and grandkids to be his primary focus, rather than his health anxiety. For Travis, "to lose ten pounds" would not be a very relevant goal, even though it is specific, measurable, and attainable. A more relevant goal for Travis was "to increase my physical stamina by taking progressively longer walks until I can walk around the lake with the family on Saturday mornings."

Timely. Set a time frame for each of your goals. Without a time limit, there's no urgency to start taking action now. It is useful to set some short-term goals (hours to weeks), midterm goals (within the next few months), and long-term goals (over a period of years). Travis was able to create a number of goals that met this requirement: "to spend thirty minutes per day on my health-anxiety homework this week" (short-term), "to increase the number of flights of stairs I climb each day by one flight per week until I can climb six floors" (midterm), and "to volunteer at the grandkids' school once a month, starting next year" (long-term).

Exercise: Make a List of Your SMART Goals

In your journal, make a list of goals for overcoming your health anxiety. Try to come up with five to ten short-, mid-, and long-term goals. You may want to refer back to the exercise "A Brighter Future," earlier in this chapter. Remember to focus on goals that are specific, measurable, attainable, relevant, and timely.

Should You Seek Treatment With a Professional?

Now that you've read this far, it seems that you are ready to make some changes and challenge your health anxiety. As we have said before, you can work through this material on your own or with a support person or professional. The choice, of course, is up to you. Many people are able to benefit significantly from self-help materials. There are, however, some situations for which you should consider including a professional in your treatment plans.

Consider consulting a professional if...

- You think you may have another, more pressing psychological disorder, such as depression or a substance-use problem.

- You find the ideas or language in this book difficult and would like someone with experience to help you go through it.

- You feel as though you need someone to help keep you accountable so that you will follow through with the homework tasks.

- You haven't had your medical complaints checked out by a doctor yet.

- You have gone through this book, worked diligently at all the exercises, and feel you are not improving (you are not moving toward your goals). But remember, you may have lived with health anxiety for many years, in which case it is unrealistic to expect it to fade completely or quickly. If you have completed all the material in this book and have practiced the exercises regularly over a period of six months or longer, you should reasonably expect to be meeting many of your short-term and midterm goals. If you aren't, it may be time to seek a professional opinion.

There are many health care providers who can help you to work on your health anxiety. These professionals may include a psychologist, psychiatrist, social worker, family doctor, or other health care professional. The most important thing is to ensure that the professional has experience in treating anxiety-related problems, and specifically health anxiety, using strategies that have been found to be effective. These strategies include the cognitive and behavioral approaches described in this book (especially in chapters 3 and 4), as well as effective medication treatments, as described in chapter 7.

In Brief...

You have outlined the toll of health anxiety on yourself and others, envisioned a better future, measured your readiness, set goals, and made a commitment to yourself. You are now ready for change. In chapter 3 you will learn more about how thoughts contribute to anxiety about your health—and how to set about changing that!

Chapter 3

Identifying and Changing Anxious Thinking

In this chapter you will begin working with your thoughts and beliefs. In chapter 1, we talked about how anxious thoughts can affect your physical sensations, direct your attention, influence what you hear and take in, and prompt your behavior. These thoughts can feed the cycle of health anxiety and can determine your experience.

Negative emotions, such as fear and anxiety, are not triggered by situations per se. Rather, they are triggered by the ways in which we interpret situations. For example, on being laid off, one worker might think, *Thank heavens! I can finally claim some of that unemployment insurance I've been socking away all these years while I hunt for a new job that I will actually enjoy.* Another person in the same circumstance might think, *Aw, hell, this is the worst thing that could possibly happen; there is no way I can cope with this right now.* Although the situation is the same in both of these examples, the two different interpretations would likely lead to very different emotional responses. Each response, one of hope versus one of despair, makes absolute sense based on each person's interpretation of the situation.

There are a number of common mistakes that almost everyone makes in their thinking. However, we often find it difficult to recognize our own errors, biases, and assumptions. There is little chance for you to make corrections if you don't know that corrections are needed! For example, if you pronounce someone's name incorrectly, chances are that you will continue doing it unless you are corrected. Once you realize your mistake, you can alter your behavior. That said, you may forget at times or slip into the old pattern, especially if you are tired, rushed, or preoccupied. The same can be true of thoughts around health anxiety; it can be easy to slip into old habits. So, what is the key to maintaining changes? The same as the key to remembering a difficult name: practice, practice, practice!

How Your Thoughts Intensify Your Health Anxiety

Thoughts play a vital role in the cycle of health anxiety, sometimes causing anxiety and sometimes serving to maintain it. The content of each thought will depend in part on the sensations or symptoms you experience, and in part on the situations in which you find yourself.

The Cycle of Health Anxiety

Emotions are comprised of three components: what we think, what we feel, and what we do (that is, our thoughts, sensations, and behaviors). For example, feelings of anxiety and fear are typically associated with predictions of doom and danger (thoughts such as *I have a serious illness*), as well as uncomfortable physical feelings (such as headaches, nausea, or palpitations) and unproductive behaviors (for example, avoiding important activities, visiting the doctor frequently, or arguing with your loved ones about minor matters). Anxiety and fear can be triggered or maintained by anxious thoughts, physical feelings, and behaviors, and the reverse also seems to be true. In other words, feelings of anxiety and fear can lead us to think in more negative ways, to feel uncomfortable sensations, and to behave fearfully.

When you notice a physical sensation or symptom (such as a head-ache, nausea, a cough, or a red patch of skin), you may start to have anxious thoughts like *I may have contracted hepatitis, This may be the beginning of something serious,* or *That looks like skin cancer.* Anxious thoughts may make the sensations themselves worse or may draw your attention to them, often leading to even more anxious thoughts, such as *There's always something wrong with me! I'll never be healthy! The world is dangerously full of contamination and disease,* or *Something is really wrong, and my doctor won't take me seriously enough.*

Anxiety-provoking thoughts, combined with a focus on your body, often lead to anxiety-related behaviors. Examples include frequent visits to the doctor's office, researching online, staying home from work, lying down, or monitoring your pulse. These behaviors often lead to some temporary relief or reassuring thoughts, such as *I'll be safe at the doctor's office* or *I will find out what is wrong, and then I will get the right treatment.* But in the long term, such behaviors tend to keep the anxiety alive. We will deal with behaviors that are associated with health anxiety in the next chapter.

Thoughts That Are Associated with Health Anxiety

There are plenty of things in life to be anxious about. That said, in the case of health anxiety, anxious thoughts tend to fall into two categories: thoughts about symptoms and thoughts about situations.

Anxious Thoughts About Symptoms

How you think about a physical sensation (such as a pounding heart) or a symptom (like a persistent cough) will often affect your level of anxiety. If you experienced a pounding heart while washing carrots, reading a magazine, or sitting in your backyard, you might think something was wrong. Your anxiety might increase. On the other hand, if you experienced this same symptom while jogging, chasing your dog around the park, or having a risqué fantasy, a pounding heart would seem pretty normal and you'd likely not experience anxious thoughts or an increase in anxiety. Coughing and choking after swallowing a bit of water the wrong way would typically not lead to much anxiety. Coughing and choking for no obvious reason could cause a spike in fear. The sensation is the same; it's the thoughts that make a difference.

Exercise: Your Automatic Thoughts About Symptoms

Think about the symptoms that typically cause you to worry about your health. You may want to refer back to the exercise "Your Physical Sensations" in chapter 1. Starting a new page in your journal, choose five or six symptoms that stand out for you; this may be because they happen often, or perhaps are especially frightening. For each symptom, write down one of the anxious thoughts that go with it. (There may be many thoughts accompanying a single symptom, but for now, write down just one.) Here are some examples:

Symptom: *Feeling a "lump" in my throat*

Thought: *I may have throat cancer, like my aunt.*

Symptom: *Feeling tired all the time*

Thought: *I have a weak immune system, leaving me open to all types of diseases and viruses.*

You will discover how important this exercise is as we progress through the book.

Anxious Thoughts About Specific Situations

Anxiety can trigger stronger, longer, or more-frightening symptoms. Your fear, discomfort, and increased attention after being in a germy situation, for example, may easily lead to having flu-like symptoms, such as a headache, nausea, clammy hands, sweating, weakness, and restlessness. These symptoms might then cause you to become even more worked up. Some situations that are common sources of stress for people who are prone to health anxiety include watching media coverage of disease outbreaks, hearing news of compromised food safety, reading about illness and disease, having a friend or family member become ill, and entering doctors' offices, medical clinics, or hospitals.

When we expect to find uncomfortable symptoms, we can often find them. If a news story, commercial, or Web page has you scanning your body and looking back at your recent health history for a certain set of symptoms, you will be much more likely to notice small changes or remember bits of evidence that fit the picture you already have in your thoughts.

Exercise: Your Automatic Thoughts About Anxiety-Provoking Situations

Think back over the past week or two about situations that you experienced as anxiety provoking and situations that caused you to worry about your health. Starting a new page in your journal, list five or six situations that stand out for you. Focus on situations that occur frequently or that are especially frightening. For each situation, write down one of the anxious thoughts that go with it. Here are some examples:

Situation: *In the waiting room at the medical clinic*

Thought: *If the doctor gives me bad news, I will absolutely fall apart.*

Situation: *Helping with hot-dog day at the school*

Thought: *These kids are carrying millions of germs and viruses that my poor immune system won't be able to deal with.*

In the next section we will work with these thoughts.

Looking at Your Thoughts

Anxiety-provoking thoughts can have a great deal of power over us. They can be incredibly difficult to interrupt, challenge, or stop. There are a number of reasons why anxious thoughts have such powerful effects, and one of them is their automatic nature.

Automatic Thoughts

Anxious thoughts are often "automatic"; that is, they are the first to pop into your mind, and may be so quick that they occur outside of awareness. You probably don't question your automatic thoughts; they seem logical and objective. When others ask, "Why would you think that?" "Doesn't that seem pretty far-fetched to you?" "Why are you worrying about something your doctor has said you don't have to worry about?" your initial reactions may have been surprise or confusion. *Why worry about these things?* A better question is how can you *not* worry? Anxious thoughts can be so automatic that you may have trouble both noticing them and identifying them as anything other than 100 percent true. When we ask people with health anxiety, "What were you thinking about when you began to notice that symptom (or decided to look up that information)?" they often respond, "Nothing." It may not be until you question your thoughts (or your television, or the information on the Internet or in the newspaper) that you notice anything negative at all.

Once you start paying attention to your thoughts (in other words, thinking about what you are thinking), it may take some time before you begin to notice specific anxious thoughts. You may have been thinking this way for so long that it has become natural. For example, if someone were to ask you what you were thinking as you made toast this morning, your first response might be, "Nothing. I was just making toast." That said, if you were to pay attention to your thoughts the next time you made toast, you might find that you were actually thinking quite a few, nearly automatic, thoughts (for example, *Take the bread out of the freezer; careful, don't knock over the frozen peas. Unwind the bag—geeze, I lost the bloody tab again. It's all freezer burned. Should I have two slices or one? I'll have two. Toast goes into the toaster, and I push the button down. I wonder if I should set the time a bit longer; limp toast is no good, and it did just come out of the freezer...*).

Automatic thoughts actually run through our minds all day long, every day. For example, when you're sitting on a bench or stool with no back, you probably aren't actively thinking that there is no back to your seat, and yet you don't lean back and fall over very often either. On some level, you are aware that your seat has no back. For you to begin challenging some of your thoughts, you must first learn to "catch" or identify them. Later in this chapter, we will provide a log just for this purpose.

Situations vs. Thoughts

At first, many people find it difficult to separate their thoughts about a situation from the objective facts of the situation. This tendency to treat our thoughts, interpretations, or beliefs as if they were hard facts is pretty normal. It's also a mental error on our part. Consider the statement "I was in the coffee shop, and everyone around me was healthy; they were all talking and smiling." In this example, there is absolutely no way the speaker could have known the health status of others in the coffee shop. The happiest-looking person could be stopping for a cup of tea before a first chemotherapy session. Meanwhile, the most miserable person you pass on the street might be incredibly healthy!

Exercise: Situations vs. Thoughts

In this exercise, try to divide each example statement into "the situation" and "the thought." The situation is limited to observable facts (such as when, where, or who). What would someone standing on the other side of a window see? The thought portion will be more subjective (such as opinions, guesses, or beliefs). Let's try an example: *I was sitting in a busy coffee shop before work, cold and tired, as usual; everyone around me was happy and healthy.*

Situation: *Sitting in a coffee shop before work*

Thoughts: *It seemed as if everyone else had it better; they all appeared healthy and happy.*

In your journal try dividing the following statements into situations and thoughts:

1. *I was sitting in my car outside the airport waiting for my wife; she had just spent hours in an airplane full of people, breathing germy, recycled air.*

2. *I was feeling flushed and took my blood pressure, which was 160/100; I've been under a dangerous amount of stress.*

3. *I watched a debate on the news about the potential pros and cons of being vaccinated against the seasonal flu; no one could provide an answer with 100 percent confidence; I'm damned if I do and damned if I don't.*

4. *I have been coughing for two weeks straight; this is more than a normal cold.*

Here is one possible set of answers:

Situation 1: *Sitting in the car*

Thought 1: *My wife will bring germs into the car with me. There's a high risk of catching something on an airplane.*

Situation 2: *Blood pressure reading of 160/100*

Thought 2: *A blood pressure reading of 160/100 is always dangerous. Stress raises my blood pressure. Stress is dangerous.*

Situation 3: *Watching the news*

Thought 3: *There is a "right" answer about the flu shot. I have not been able to find the right answer. I may make the wrong choice, and that would be dangerous.*

Situation 4: *Experiencing a two-week-long bout of coughing*

Thought 4: *Coughing for two weeks means the cough must be due to something more serious than a cold.*

Now that you have an idea of the types of situations in your life that create thoughts around health anxiety, you are ready to take the next step.

Types of Biased Thinking

There are many different types of automatic thoughts. Most of the time, they are useful mental shortcuts, but at other times, they lead us to erroneous conclusions. If you are like most people, you probably overestimate the likelihood of bad things happening, misinterpret situations as being more catastrophic than they are, and pay more attention to information that confirms your beliefs than that which counters them. The following sections discuss these common thinking errors that can contribute to anxiety.

Errors in Estimating Probability

Probability overestimation involves assuming that an event or outcome is more likely than it really is. For example, sometimes Heather had a strong belief that she had undiagnosed bacterial meningitis. Heather believed that the likelihood that she had or would develop bacterial meningitis was about 1 in 100. In fact, the chances are a lot less, somewhere between 1 in 33,000 and 1 in 100,000. She overestimated her risk by between 330 and 1,000 percent. Another person might think *Using cutlery in restaurants is often a high-risk behavior,* although most people eat from restaurant cutlery and never experience any ill effects. The thought that it's often risky is an example of an overestimation.

The flip side of overestimation is underestimation, and people with health anxiety tend to do this as well. In addition to overestimating unlikely possibilities for a cough (lung cancer, acute respiratory distress syndrome, emphysema), the most likely candidates (dry air, the common cold, allergies) are often underestimated. Are there any unlikely illnesses or outcomes that you have, at times, thought were likely suspects? What about more likely scenarios that you doubted or discounted?

Probability overestimations and underestimations can occur when we misinterpret the meaning of a particular event or situation. For example, consider a man who is already anxious about his work situation, who rushes into the office five minutes late after being caught in traffic and finds a note on his desk asking him to drop by his boss's office. He might believe that his supervisor came to his office, found out he was late, and now is about to fire him. He might become caught up in a chain of negative thoughts that ends up with images of his wife taking the kids and leaving, the house being foreclosed, and his parents being ejected from their nursing home. You can imagine the state that our anxious person might be in when he finally gathers up the courage to go to his employer's office! At that point it doesn't matter how mistaken he is; his anxiety will have taken over because of how he interpreted the meaning of the note his boss had left.

People with health anxiety tend to misinterpret the meaning of ambiguous information as possibly indicating a risk of harm or disease. For example, Jeanne found a note about pandemic planning in her son's backpack. She immediately thought that the school had to know something she didn't, that her son was in imminent danger, and that the whole family would likely become seriously ill.

Catastrophic Thinking

When people engage in catastrophic thinking, they mistakenly overestimate how horrible an outcome would be if it were to occur, and they underestimate their ability to cope with it. They may assume that an outcome is more important or meaningful than it really is. Examples of catastrophic thoughts include:

- *It would be a disaster if I were to catch a cold.*

- *I couldn't possibly cope if I were to throw up.*

- *If my child were to get sick, I don't think I could handle it.*

- *It would be terrible if I couldn't see my doctor when I feel anxious.*

Although these thoughts would likely be anxiety provoking for someone who experiences high levels of health anxiety, each of these situations would likely be more manageable than they seem.

Confirmation Biases

The term *confirmation bias* refers to a common tendency we have to search for, interpret, and remember information in a way that confirms our own preconceptions. People do not purposely go out of their way to think in a biased fashion and often don't even know they are doing it. People who are afraid to fly in airplanes, for example, are often acutely aware of accidents and may be able to recite a list of recent air disasters. They may remember articles about safety lapses and news programs about crashes. This is called *selective memory*, because they remember information that confirms their beliefs more easily than they recall disconfirming information. All of this information is consistent with the belief that air travel is inherently and extremely dangerous. Flights that go well are ignored, forgotten, or discounted.

People with health anxiety can, at times, selectively remember a small and specific sliver of information (for example, that the doctor started his good news about your test results with, "Now, no test is completely infallible, but..."). You may also doubt whether your memory of a given situation, conversation, or set of information is accurate (for example, *I thought the doctor said that the rash should go away in a week and that I didn't need to see her again, but what if I'm wrong? Perhaps she said that if the rash completely goes away, I don't have to come back. Maybe she needs to see me again if it hasn't totally cleared.*).

The confirmation bias is particularly strong when issues are highly personally significant. This makes sense when we think about sensations or symptoms. You most likely notice, worry about, and remember when sensations and symptoms are present, but may fail to notice when they are absent. This is referred to as *selective attention*. The times your health fears have been borne out (for example, the one time you thought you had food poisoning, and you were right) will be remembered and used as evidence to support future anxious thoughts, whereas the dozens, hundreds, or thousands of times your fears were unfounded (such as all the times a headache did *not* turn out to be anything serious, a high blood pressure reading did *not* lead to a stroke, or going to the store did *not* lead to a panic attack) will not be given equal weight. Essentially, when people are anxious or afraid, they tend to pay more attention to information that confirms their anxious thoughts than to information that challenges or disconfirms them.

Exercise: Identifying Biases

The following types of thoughts often seem more like facts than errors in thinking. Take a moment to see if you can identify instances of (a) probability overestimations or underestimations, (b) catastrophic thinking, and (c) confirmation biases (for example, selective memory and attention). More than one may fit.

1. *This cough is surely a sign of lung cancer.*

2. *If my daughter gets sick, I won't be able to handle it.*

3. *I specifically remember that the nurse said people have allergic reactions to this vaccination.*

4. *Every article about being overweight warns of diabetes and heart disease.*

5. *There is no harmless explanation for such awful headaches.*

6. *If my blood pressure rises, I will have a stroke and die.*

7. *My pulse is always thready.*

8. *These chiropractic exercises leave me stiff and sore. They must be bad for my back.*

Answer Key:

1. Probability overestimation

2. Catastrophic thinking

3. Confirmation bias

4. Confirmation bias

5. Probability underestimation

6. Catastrophic thinking

7. Confirmation bias

8. Probability overestimation

Are You Any Less Prone Than Others to Having Thinking Errors?

In spite of all we have just discussed about biases in thinking, attention, and memory, it would be pretty normal for you to think, *I can see how others with health anxiety make those kinds of errors, but I don't make those kinds of mistakes. I'm just more vigilant* (or *more sensitive, more aware, more knowledgeable, more in tune with my body, more prone to illness,* and so on) *than most people.* It's all well and good for us to point out all the potential mistakes other people with health anxiety make, but what about you? Many people with anxiety think that their situation is somehow different and that their thoughts are not unduly influenced by anxiety.

Is it possible that people with health anxiety are just better at monitoring and judging their physiological sensations than those without health anxiety? This does not seem to be the case. People who worry about their health, monitor their sensations, or pay a great deal of attention to illness are no better at judging the state of their health or the seriousness of a threat than anyone else (Salkovskis, Warwick, and Deale 2003). Although it may seem as if those around you are too lax in attending to their bodies or are not concerned enough about illness and disease, they are, in fact, behaving quite adaptively, in that they are adjusting to their environments constructively.

Tracking Your Thoughts

The very act of recording a behavior can lead to a change in the frequency of the behavior. For example, people who are asked to track their smoking habits tend to smoke less than they did before they began documenting where, when, and how often they smoked (Karoly and Doyle 1975). Similarly, tracking weight, calories, meals, snacks, and drinks can lead to a decrease in the number of calories consumed (Baker and Kirschenbaum 1993). Recording the situation and your thoughts during incidents in which you feel angry enough to punch someone in the nose can change your response, making you less likely to lash out. To reduce your health anxiety, it will be important for you to identify, challenge, and change your thoughts around health anxiety. Recording your thoughts is the first step in this process.

Thoughts Are Hypotheses

Notice that so far, nowhere have we said that all your thoughts and worries about your health are wrong. Nor did we say they are all over-blown, misinterpretations, or excessive. Many people with health anxiety have real health concerns. We'll never ask you to stop worrying about your health entirely, to ignore all symptoms, or to just think positively.

All thoughts, related to health anxiety or not, are just that: thoughts (or ideas, guesses, or hypotheses). Often our beliefs are accurate. For example, when we turn on the faucet, we expect water; we assume that a stove costs more than a blender; we imagine that the dry cleaner knows more about cleaning fabric than we do. It's no wonder then that anxious thoughts seem to be true; many of our thoughts *are* true.

Thoughts around health anxiety can be so powerful that they seem beyond question. When we begin to monitor, document, and take a hard look at our thoughts, they are often not as true as they first seem. Let's take a common anxiety-provoking thought around health: *This* _____ (insert any symptom you commonly worry about) *is undoubtedly a sign of a serious illness or disease.* This negative and automatic thought cannot, strictly speaking, always be true. Virtually every symptom, whether it be a headache, bowel changes, shaky hands, or a lump, can be explained in many different ways. This is true for both common and uncommon symptoms. Often, the explanation is innocuous.

However, the negative thought may certainly seem true. Believing that something is true—and having strong emotions along with that belief—doesn't make it so. Many people with health anxiety occasionally (or often) have thoughts such as *I know I'm sick, Dangerous germs are everywhere, The doctor didn't understand me, The tests are wrong* (or *incomplete* or *inconclusive*), *I am more illness prone than other people, No one is taking me seriously,* or *I am going to die.* Does any of this sound familiar? The next step in challenging your health anxiety is for you to start to figure out which of your anxious thoughts are true and which merely seem true. To do this, you need to begin recording your anxiety-provoking thoughts around health. In the next several sections, you will learn how to compile evidence for and against the thoughts, and then propose a thought that takes all the evidence into account.

When to Record Your Thoughts

Recording behaviors like cigarette smoking or food intake is pretty straightforward. Recording thoughts, on the other hand, can be challenging, because they are often so automatic that they go unnoticed. There are a few signs you can watch for. One indication that it might be a good idea to record your thoughts is if you notice a distinct and negative change in your mood. If you find yourself feeling anxious, apprehensive, afraid, panicky, sad, or hopeless, for example, your thoughts may be related to health anxiety.

Other situations in which it would be useful to record your thoughts include: being exposed to worrisome health information (such as a news story); finding yourself seeking health information (such as researching a symptom online); feeling ill; noticing that someone close to you is ill; receiving comments from other people that you are worrying too much; or doing things that reflect anxiety about your health (for example, taking your pulse, checking your stool, taking megadoses of vitamins). There is a strong possibility that in situations such as these, some of your thoughts are related to health anxiety. It is these thoughts that you should notice and then write down.

Questions to Help Identify Thoughts That Contribute to Health Anxiety

In the next exercise, we'll help you to become more familiar with your anxious thoughts. If it has been a while since you first started this chapter, take a few minutes to review the material, reminding yourself of what to look for. You know that some of your anxiety-provoking thoughts and predictions may be automatic and hard to catch. To identify what types of anxiety-provoking, health-related thoughts affect you, you will have to pay close attention. Here are some questions to help you identify these thoughts:

▣ *What am I thinking right now?*

▣ *What am I afraid might happen? Then what?*

▣ *Are there any frightening images in my mind?*

▣ *What happened just before I got anxious?*

▣ *What was I thinking just before I got anxious?*

Exercise: Completing Anxiety Thought Records

Anxiety thought records may look a bit complicated until you get the hang of it. Don't worry; we're going to work through this important skill in several steps. After some practice this will become much easier. Do your best to complete at least one anxiety thought record each day. The thought record will be your tool for identifying anxiety-provoking thoughts and predictions, as well as the feelings they lead to. They will be an avenue for you to look at alternative thoughts and predictions, evidence regarding your thoughts, and realistic conclusions. Often, this process will lead to a change in the intensity of the emotion you are feeling. You can either develop your own record or copy the one in this book. Each thought record can take a fair amount of space, so you'll likely want a whole page for each. On the next page is a blank anxiety thought record for copying.

Anxiety Thought Record

Day and time	Situation	Anxiety-provoking thoughts and predictions	Anxiety before (0–100)	Alternative thoughts	Evidence and realistic conclusions	Anxiety after (0–100)

For now, just complete the first four columns. In the first column, begin by writing the day and time. In the second column, briefly note the facts of the situation (if you write more than a few words here, you are probably recording a thought rather than the situation). Think about how someone else would describe the situation if they were looking at a photo of it or looking at you through a window. In the third column, record your anxious thoughts and predictions. Remember, earlier in this chapter, we went over some questions to ask yourself to help identify the anxious thoughts if you get stuck.

Once you have written down all the thoughts you can think of, double-check to see if any are missing. Is there some anxiety you are experiencing that you haven't described a thought for? If so, add this information now. Don't screen your answers even if you feel that some of your thoughts seem "silly" or don't make sense logically. If all of your thoughts were 100 percent objective and reasonable, you probably wouldn't be reading this book! In the fourth column, record your level of anxiety from 0 (no anxiety at all) to 100 (anxious feelings as strong as you can imagine).

Again, just focus on the first four columns for now, and try to complete at least one anxiety thought record every day. A sample record with just the first four columns completed is provided next. Once you have completed the first four columns for five thought records, move on to the next section in this chapter.

Sample Completed Anxiety Thought Record (First Four Columns Only)			
Day and time	**Situation**	**Anxiety-provoking thoughts and predictions**	**Anxiety before (0–100)**
January 9/ 8:20 a.m.	Parked outside the airport to pick up my wife	*Airplanes are full of dangerous germs! I'll get sick with the flu or something worse.* *I have a weak immune system.* *I'll get sick because my wife dragged these germs into my car, and it will drive a wedge between us.* *She should have taken a cab. She knows I'll be anxious when she carries all those germs into my car.* *My wife doesn't care if I get sick.* *Other spouses go into the airport to meet their partners, but I'm too afraid.*	85

Challenging Anxious Thoughts

Until now, this chapter has focused on how thoughts and predictions related to health anxiety can make us experience the world in a biased way. When we're anxious, worried, or afraid, thoughts may seem true, even though they may or may not be true. In this section, you will focus on alternative thoughts and predictions, collecting evidence, and determining if your thoughts are, in fact, true. You may find that they're not as true as you initially thought. We are not saying that all of your anxious thoughts are false. For example, if you always become nauseous and vomit when you have a headache, then the thought *I'm going to vomit* next time you have a headache is probably a realistic one. However, if you can remember times when you had a headache and didn't vomit, then that negative thought would not be 100 percent true. This section will teach you to think about and evaluate alternatives to your thoughts, rather than simply assume that your thoughts are true.

Questions to Challenge Anxious Thoughts

The rest of this chapter will focus on completing the remaining three columns of the anxiety thought record. At first, it may be difficult to identify alternative thoughts and predictions (the fifth column). The following questions will help you challenge negative thoughts and will come in handy as you complete the fifth and sixth columns on the thought record:

- *How do I know this is true?*

- *Have I had experiences in which my thought or prediction didn't come true?*

- *Is my anxious thought 100 percent true, 100 percent of the time?*

- *What is the realistic probability that this thought or prediction will come true?*

- *Have I been in this type of situation before? What happened?*

- *If this has happened before, what's different now?*

- *What are other possible explanations for the symptoms I am experiencing?*

- *If the worst thing happened, how bad would it really be?*

- *How could I cope with the situation if it were to come true?*

- *What would I say if a friend were having this worry?*

- *What might a friend, relative, or significant other without significant health anxiety think if the person were in my situation?*

Not all of these questions will be useful for every one of your anxiety-related thoughts. For example, if you were thinking *I'm going to die*, asking yourself *If the worst thing happened, how bad would it really be?* would not be useful. Instead, a more useful question might be *What is the realistic probability that this thought or prediction will come true?* On the other hand, if your anxious prediction were *I'm going to catch a cold*, then *How bad would that really be?* might be a very useful question.

Collecting Evidence

In addition to helping you devise alternative thoughts (the fifth column), asking yourself these important questions will provide you with key evidence concerning your thoughts and predictions. This will include evidence that supports your anxious thoughts and that which contradicts them (the sixth column). Without evidence, it's impossible to evaluate the accuracy of your thoughts. Imagine that you're helping to choose someone in your workplace to be employee of the year. Imagine that Darius says, "I am the best salesman *ever!*" Would you believe it? Would you automatically sign him up for the award and consider the job done? Why not? How would you evaluate Darius's assertion? You would probably ask him for evidence. As would a scientist, lawyer, or judge, you might say, "Prove it."

Darius's answer would help you determine whether his assertion that he is the best is, in fact, correct. Imagine if he responded with, "I have had the highest sales in the branch for the last four years and the highest sales in the whole company for the past two years; also, seven of my last eight trainees have outperformed their colleagues each quarter, and *Salesperson Monthly* did a feature article on me; oh, and here's a photo of me on the cover, wearing our company shirt." Then you might be convinced that Darius's claim was true. You might send the plaque out that day to be engraved with his name!

On the other hand, if Darius had said, "Well, I'm the best salesman just because I am," you might be a little less convinced. You also might start looking to other employees as potential award recipients. Thoughts related to health anxiety may seem true "just because." You may believe they're true simply because you don't know differently or because you've always thought this way.

In the next exercise, you will begin to challenge your anxious thoughts. At first, it may be helpful to imagine that your thoughts are "trying to convince you" that they are correct. As would a scientist, lawyer, or judge, you will need to ask challenging questions. Tell your anxiety to prove it! Go back to your earlier thought records with the first four columns completed. If you haven't filled them in yet, give yourself a few days to complete the forms, as described earlier. It isn't enough to just try this in your head. Developing alternative thoughts is a skill that needs to be learned over time, just like playing the piano or completing math problems. Completing the process on paper is a helpful way of practicing this skill, especially at the beginning. After some practice, you will be able to do this in your head, right when the anxiety hits.

Exercise: Completing Your Anxiety Thought Records

When you look back at your thought records, you will probably find that you were able to come up with a number of negative thoughts in each situation. If you had difficulty with this, go back to the section "Questions to Help Identify Thoughts That Contribute to Health Anxiety" and see if you can identify a few more thoughts for each situation.

When we look at people's thought records, often there is one thought or prediction that is most responsible for the anxiety reported. These scariest thoughts, the ones that make your health anxiety spike, are thoughts like *I may die from a heart attack, like my dad* or *These headaches are signs of a brain tumor*, and they affect the way you feel. Think of a time when you felt really bad and ask yourself, *What was I thinking?*

Now, look back on the thoughts you recorded in your four-column entries. Which thoughts were really driving your feelings? Circle, underline, or highlight the driving thought for each thought record you started. The next three columns will be completed in reference to this most intense thought or prediction. In the fifth column, record some alternative, nonanxious ways of thinking about the situation. If you are able to develop alternatives to the most urgent, pressing, or distressing thought, and come to a realistic conclusion, there is a good chance that your anxiety will decrease.

In the sixth column, list evidence that you believe supports your anxious thought and evidence that you believe contradicts it. Once you have alternative thoughts and predictions as well as evidence, record a more realistic or balanced conclusion, based on the evidence. Based on your more balanced conclusion, rate your anxiety again in the seventh column. Has the intensity of your anxiety changed? If you have come up with a more objective, logical, believable thought, your feelings should reflect this. Don't expect that you will suddenly go from an anxiety rating of 85 to feeling no anxiety at all. However, if you have considered a full range of possible interpretations and thoughts, your negative emotions should be less intense. Complete at least one thought record every day.

On the next page is a sample of a fully completed anxiety thought record.

Sample Completed Anxiety Thought Record

Day and time	Situation	Anxiety-provoking thoughts and predictions	Anxiety before (0–100)	Alternative thoughts	Evidence and realistic conclusions	Anxiety after (0–100)
January 9/ 8:20 a.m.	Parked outside the airport to pick up my wife	Airplanes are full of dangerous germs! I'll get sick with the flu or something worse. I have a weak immune system. I'll get sick because my wife dragged these germs into my car, and it will drive a wedge between us. She should have taken a cab. She knows I'll be anxious when she carries all those germs into my car. **My wife doesn't care if I get sick.** Other spouses go into the airport to meet their partners, but I'm too afraid.	85	Maybe she missed me and that's why she asked me to pick her up. My wife wants a ride home from me because it is cheaper and easier than taking a cab. Many people do not worry about germs as much as I do, and most of them seem perfectly healthy. My wife does not worry about germs as I do; she probably does not consider getting in the car with me to be a threat. Flying is likely not as germy as I think.	She didn't call a cab, even though it would have been safer for me than filling my car with germs. On the other hand, she has flown before, and I have never actually gotten sick from driving her home. My wife bought this book to help me. When I was home sick with the flu, she went out for lunch with her mother—but she also went out and bought me soup, tissues, and aspirin. Realistic conclusion: Although I find it frightening, my wife's asking me for a ride home does not mean she doesn't care about my health, and it does not mean I will get sick.	40

Troubleshooting

This section includes solutions to a few common challenges that often arise when using the cognitive strategies described in this chapter.

Problem:	*I have difficulty pinpointing my anxious thoughts.*
Solution:	• Ask yourself the "Questions to Help Identify Thoughts That Contribute to Health Anxiety."
Problem:	*I have difficulty finding evidence against my anxious thoughts.*
Solutions:	• Ask yourself the "Questions to Challenge Anxious Thoughts." • Ask someone else how they might view the situation. • View the situation as a scientist, lawyer, or judge might. • If you still cannot come up with a speck of evidence questioning the 100 percent truth of your anxious thought, maybe it is correct.
Problem:	*I completed an anxiety thought record, but the intensity of my anxiety did not change.*
Solution:	• You may not believe your own alternative thoughts and realistic conclusion. Double-check: Did you challenge the most pressing thought? Is there an underlying thought or prediction you may have missed? If so, go through a new record, challenging the new thought.

In Brief...

In this chapter you learned how your thoughts can make you feel worse, about common types of anxious thinking, and about situations in which anxious thinking likely plays a role. You learned how to identify your anxiety-provoking thoughts and predictions related to health and began to master the process of changing them. The ability to shift anxious thinking takes regular practice before it becomes natural. As you work your way through the rest of this book, continue to complete at least one anxiety thought record each day, or complete one whenever you have an episode of anxiety over your health. In chapter 4 you will work on another vital skill for dealing with health anxiety: changing your typical patterns of anxious behavior.

Chapter 4

Identifying and Changing Anxious Behaviors

Think back to a time in your life when you had an irrational fear of some specific object or situation that no longer troubles you today. For example, were you frightened of clowns as a young child? Or were you very nervous the first few times you dated your current partner? Did you experience fear when skiing for the first time, or swimming or driving? Can you think of a situation or object that once frightened you, but no longer does? If so, how did you get over your fear? Did you do something specific that led you to become more comfortable?

Now, imagine that you have a close friend, Lili, who has an extreme fear of cats. She avoids cats at all cost, and even avoids places where she might see a cat (such as visiting friends who have cats, walking by a pet store, and going for a stroll in her neighborhood). Before Lili leaves home, she has her husband check to see if there are any cats nearby. If there is a cat outside her house, her husband must chase the cat away before Lili will walk to her car. Lili's fear goes back more than twenty years and has not improved at all. Why do you think Lili's fear has stayed the same for so long? What might Lili be doing (unintentionally) to keep her fear alive? What strategies might you recommend for Lili to get over her fear?

These scenarios are meant to help you consider possible behaviors that maintain fear over time, as well as strategies you can use to reduce fear and anxiety. As you may have guessed, avoiding feared situations is likely to keep fear alive over the long term, whereas facing your fears is a powerful way to reduce them. In fact, a 1999 report on mental health by the Surgeon General of the United States concluded that a "critical element of therapy is to increase exposure to the stimuli or situations that provoke anxiety" (U.S. Department of Health and Human Services 1999, 241). Furthermore, hundreds of studies going back more than a half century have shown that the more often we face our fears, the easier it becomes to do the things that frighten us (Moscovitch, Antony, and Swinson 2009).

In other words, if you did overcome a fear in the past, there is a good chance that forcing yourself to do the things you feared is what led to a reduction in your fear. In the same way, spending more time around cats would probably reduce Lili's fear. This chapter will help you to apply these principles to your own health anxiety, and will teach you strategies for reducing your fear by changing your behaviors.

Behaviors That Contribute to Health Anxiety

In chapter 3, we discussed how your beliefs influence whether you experience anxiety in specific situations. For example, if you believe that a racing heart is a sign of a heart attack, you will probably experience anxiety when your heart races, even if your racing heart has a perfectly harmless explanation (for example, perhaps you just ran up a flight of stairs, you're feeling anxious, or you drank too much coffee). If exaggerated anxious beliefs are responsible for maintaining your feelings of anxiety, you may wonder why your anxious beliefs don't naturally change over time, as you observe over and over again that they don't come true. The answer has to do with how you respond to your thoughts—in other words, your behaviors. If you avoid the situations you fear, you never learn that the situations are in fact safe, and your anxious thoughts continue. Similarly, if you do things to protect yourself from possible harm (even though there is no real danger), you never learn that your safety behaviors are unnecessary, again keeping your anxious thoughts from being challenged. We will now consider the role of safety behaviors and avoidance in more detail.

Safety Behaviors

Safety behaviors are actions that we take to protect ourselves from possible harm or to feel safe in the situations we fear. Examples of safety behaviors people with elevated health anxiety often use include:

- Seeking reassurance from family members and friends, including such examples as asking them about the meaning of your symptoms ("I'm feeling dizzy; why do you think that is?"), comparing your symptoms to theirs ("I have a sharp pain behind my eyes. Do you ever get that feeling?"), and asking them to check your symptoms ("Do you think this mark on my arm might be cancer?")

- Seeking reassurance from doctors

- Seeking reassurance from other sources, such as medical books, the Internet, or the media (for example, medical television shows)

- Requesting frequent, unnecessary medical tests

- Monitoring physical symptoms, such as pain, racing heart, dizziness, or blurred vision

- Checking for physical changes in your body, such as increased blood pressure; changes in weight; or unusual sores, lumps, or rashes

- Following rigid rules about food (for example, eating broccoli every day based on media reports that it reduces the risk of cancer)

- Following overly rigid rules about exercise and other health behaviors

- Avoiding all sun exposure to prevent skin cancer

- Washing your hands dozens of times each day to avoid getting sick

In moderation, many of these behaviors are helpful. For example, there is nothing wrong with striving for a balanced diet, exercising regularly, and seeing your doctor for an annual checkup. The behaviors on this list are a problem only when they occur excessively. When taken to the extreme, these behaviors are unnecessary, time consuming, expensive, and possibly even dangerous. In addition, they help to maintain your anxiety. Engaging in these behaviors can strengthen your belief that they are necessary, in much the same way that having her husband check for cats reinforced Lili's belief that she needed him to do this.

Exercise: Identifying Safety Behaviors

In your journal, make a list of safety behaviors you use to reduce your anxiety, to check for signs that you may be ill, or to prevent yourself from getting sick. For each safety behavior, make a note of how often you use it and how much time it takes up. Safety behaviors that are most problematic are those that occur frequently, take up a lot of time, or interfere significantly in your day-to-day life. It may be helpful to refer back to the list of behaviors that contribute to your health anxiety you prepared in chapter 1.

Avoidance

It is perfectly natural to avoid situations that trigger fear and anxiety. We do this to protect ourselves from possible harm. In fact, avoidance makes perfect sense in many situations. For example, most people would avoid opening the front door if they heard gunshots in front of their homes. Similarly, many people (wisely) avoid spending time with acquaintances who constantly put them down. However, avoidance is not always helpful, particularly in situations where there is no realistic threat. Like safety behaviors, avoidance can help to decrease anxiety and fear in the short term. However, avoiding feared stimuli keeps your fear alive over the long term.

There are three general types of avoidance that can contribute to anxiety over time. The first is *situational avoidance*, which involves avoiding external objects, places, or situations. Examples of situations that people with health anxiety may avoid include:

- Seeing a doctor for a checkup or procedure

- Undergoing medical tests

- Visiting a friend in the hospital

- Visiting a clinic that specializes in treating a feared disease (for example, a cancer clinic)

- Reading about health issues in books or on the Web

- Watching medical shows on television

- Talking to others about health, illness, or a particular feared disease

- Touching objects that you believe may be contaminated (for example, using public restrooms)

- Eating foods that you believe may lead to illness (for example, eating meat or drinking tap water)

- Exposing yourself to situations involving death (for example, attending a funeral, reading obituaries)

A second type of avoidance that is common among people with heightened health anxiety is *symptom avoidance*, which refers to avoidance of feared physical sensations, such as racing heart, dizziness, or breathlessness. People who are anxious about their health often experience anxiety in response to physical symptoms that they believe to be dangerous. For example, dizziness is likely to be anxiety provoking if it is misinterpreted as a sign of stroke. A headache may be terrifying if it is mistaken for a brain tumor. Although people with health anxiety often scan their bodies for the symptoms they fear, they may also go out of their way to avoid experiencing feared symptoms. Examples of symptom avoidance include:

- Avoiding foods that trigger feared symptoms such as sweating (spicy foods) or racing heart (coffee)

- Avoiding physical exercise, sports, sex, or other arousing activities

- Avoiding places that are hot and stuffy

- Avoiding stressful situations that trigger symptoms of physical arousal

- Avoiding scary movies, conflict, celebrations, or other activities that trigger strong emotions

A third type of avoidance is *cognitive avoidance,* which involves avoiding thoughts or images that trigger anxiety. People who experience high levels of anxiety may believe that their anxiety-provoking thoughts are dangerous. For example, a person with health anxiety may hold the belief that thinking about a heart attack may trigger one. Or someone might worry about becoming overwhelmed or losing control unless she blocks all thoughts of illness from entering consciousness (perhaps through distraction or other thought-suppression methods). Although the suppression of feared thoughts may help for a short time, these efforts often cause thoughts to become more distressing afterward and may even lead to increases in the frequency of feared thoughts.

Exercise: Identifying Avoidance Behaviors

In your journal, make lists of (1) objects, places, or situations you avoid; (2) sensations you avoid; and (3) thoughts or images you try to avoid or suppress. Later, this information will be useful when it comes time to develop exposure practices.

Guidelines for Preventing Safety Behaviors

Earlier in this chapter, you generated a list of safety behaviors: things you do to feel more comfortable when anxiety strikes. In many ways, safety behaviors for people with excessive health anxiety serve a function similar to the function drugs or alcohol perform for a person with an addiction. Safety behaviors temporarily reduce your discomfort, but as long as you keep doing them, your desire to use these behaviors keeps coming back and may even get stronger over time. Just as the drug abuser must reduce or stop using drugs in order to overcome his addiction, it's important that you reduce or eliminate your use of safety behaviors to see a reduction in your health anxiety.

You can do this in one of two ways. The first method is *complete response prevention*, which involves eliminating the safety behavior completely. For example, if you frequently seek reassurance from your family or visit your doctor every week, you would stop these behaviors entirely. An advantage of complete response prevention is that you quickly learn to function without relying on safety behaviors, and you soon notice a sharp drop in anxiety.

A second method is *gradual response prevention*, which involves eliminating the safety behavior in steps. For example, you might reduce the frequency of checking your body for marks on your skin by 20 percent the first week, another 20 percent the second week, another 20 percent the third week, and so on until you finally reach a point where you no longer need to check. Another example of gradual response prevention involves delaying safety behaviors. For example, rather than check the Internet for reassurance about a symptom as soon as the urge occurs, you could delay checking for two hours and then reevaluate your urge to check. At that point, the urge to check may have passed. If it is still overwhelming, you can decide then whether to act on it or to delay further. Over time, you might increase the length of the delay gradually until you reach a point where the safety behavior has been eliminated entirely.

Ideally, we recommend that you cut out your safety behaviors entirely. Complete response prevention is likely to lead to changes in anxiety more quickly than a more gradual approach. On the other hand, if complete response prevention is too frightening, then reducing your safety behaviors gradually is an excellent alternative. Regardless of which approach you take, preventing your safety behaviors will probably be difficult. First, some safety behaviors are automatic, like habits. You may even be unaware that you're using a safety behavior, perhaps until after it's too late. Monitoring your use of safety behaviors in your journal will help to make you more aware of them. Second, the urge to seek reassurance or to use other safety behaviors is sometimes overwhelming—it may even feel like a matter of life and death! There are a number of strategies you can use to deal with overwhelming urges to use your safety behaviors:

- Don't fight your feelings of anxiety. Just wait out the urge to complete your safety behavior. Often, the urge is strongest at the beginning and dissipates over time. Fighting your anxiety keeps it alive for longer.

- Get involved in some other activity. For example, watch a favorite movie or go for a walk rather than focus on your urge to complete the behavior.

- Phone a friend, seek support from your partner, or talk to a close family member (without using this contact to seek reassurance). Social support can be an effective way to cope with anxiety.

- Challenge the thoughts and predictions that contribute to your anxiety, by examining the evidence or completing a thought record (see chapter 3).

- Meditate, slow down your breathing, or try some muscle relaxation exercises (see chapter 6).

- Reward yourself for not using safety behaviors. For example, plan a nice dinner out each week you are able to get through without using your safety behaviors.

Don't expect your response prevention efforts to go perfectly. You may find that you slip back a bit for every few steps you move forward. Despite your best efforts, you may not always be able to stop yourself from visiting your doctor, checking your blood pressure, or using some other safety behaviors. When this happens, it will be important not to get down on yourself. Small slips are normal. Just put them behind you and move on.

Exercise: Preventing Safety Behaviors

In your journal, keep track of your efforts to resist completing safety behaviors. Each time you get the urge to monitor a symptom, seek reassurance, check the Internet, book an appointment with your doctor, or complete some other safety behavior, resist the urge. Make a note of:

1. The date and time

2. Which safety behavior you feel compelled to complete

3. The intensity of the urge to complete the behavior, using a scale from 0 (no urge at all) to 100 (extremely strong urge)

4. How long it took your anxiety to subside without using the safety behavior

5. Whether you ended up giving in to the urge and completing your safety behavior

You may find it easiest to develop a form with five columns to track these details (see the following example). Continue this exercise throughout your treatment. Monitoring your checking, reassurance seeking, and related safety behaviors will help you to reduce your reliance on them.

Safety Behavior Tracking Form				
Date/Time	Safety Behavior	Urge Intensity (0–100)	Duration of Urge	Completed Safety Behavior?
December 17/ 2:00 p.m.	Check blood pressure	98	60 minutes	No

When to See Your Doctor

Everyone has symptoms from time to time that warrant a visit to the doctor. At what point should you see your doctor? We recommend that you meet with your family physician up front to explain that you are trying to reduce your anxiety about health and that your program involves eliminating unnecessary medical visits. Then ask your doctor for suggestions regarding how to decide whether an office visit is a good idea. The answer to this question is not always simple, and will depend on such factors as your health history, age, risk factors (for example, being overweight or having a family history of cancer), the type of symptom you are experiencing, and how long the symptom has lasted. Often, it is useful to rely on a "two-week rule" (Furer, Walker, and Stein 2007). Many symptoms, including aches and pains, rashes, colds, and other minor ailments, clear up on their own within a week or two.

If your health is fairly good, you have few risk factors, and the types of symptoms you experience are similar to those you have experienced in the past, it is probably fine not to see your doctor. On the other hand, if a symptom is new, particularly severe, or doesn't go away on its own, it may be worth checking out. Similarly, it might make sense to check out symptoms of a particular illness sooner rather than later if you have an increased risk for developing that illness (for example, if you have a history of cancer or heart disease). One benefit of visiting your doctor less frequently is that she will likely take your symptoms more seriously when you do come in for a visit! Chapter 5 includes additional suggestions for deciding whether to visit your doctor.

Guidelines for Effective Exposure

As discussed in the previous section, reducing your use of safety behaviors is one method for learning that you can cope with your feelings of anxiety and that you don't have to constantly protect yourself from possible threats. Another important method for reducing fear is confronting feared situations rather than avoiding them. This method is often referred to as *exposure therapy*, since it involves exposing yourself to situations that you typically avoid. Usually, exposure therapy is used in combination with the response prevention strategies for reducing safety behaviors (discussed earlier).

How you undertake exposure is important for ensuring that you obtain the outcome you want. Not all exposure is therapeutic. For example, if you were terrified of snakes and someone threw a snake at you, your fear would probably get worse rather than better. For exposure to be helpful, there are a number of guidelines you need to consider as you carry out your practices. These guidelines are described next.

Exposures Should Be Predictable and Under Your Control

Exposure is most effective when it is *predictable* (in other words, you know what is likely to happen during the practice and when it will happen) and when you are in *control* (that is, you are in charge of when the practice begins, what happens during the practice, and when it ends). For example, if you are scheduled to undergo a feared medical test, it may be helpful to find out what the procedure involves and how long you are likely to have to wait for the results. You should never be tricked or forced into doing something you haven't agreed to do. Also, the possibility of surprises should be minimized during exposure practices. Reading the obituaries each day (if this is a situation you fear) would be a good example of an exposure that is predictable and under your control.

Design Exposures to Test Specific Predictions

Chapter 3 discussed the importance of viewing your anxious predictions as hypotheses rather than facts. Just as scientists conduct experiments to investigate whether their hypotheses are true, you can use your exposure practices to test the accuracy of your beliefs. For example, if you are convinced that running on a treadmill will trigger a heart attack (even though your doctor says you are in fine health), you can design exposure practices that involve running on a treadmill to test your prediction and learn that your assumption isn't true.

In some cases, it may be impossible to design exposures to test a particular thought. For example, if you believe that reducing your hand washing from fifty times a day to five times a day will increase your chances of developing cancer in the future, it may take years to find out whether your belief is true. Still, reducing your hand washing is likely to help reduce your fear over time (though initially it will likely increase your fear).

Exposures Should Be Gradual

For exposure to be effective, it is important to carry out practices that arouse fear. Exposures are akin to exercise in this way—if you don't feel anything, the task may be too easy. However, you don't need to start off with the most frightening practices you can imagine. Rather, we recommend starting with more manageable practices and working up to more challenging ones. The quicker you move on to more difficult practices, the more discomfort you will experience, but the quicker you will overcome your fear. We recommend that you try to challenge yourself, but don't worry if a particular task is too difficult. You can work up to it gradually. An *exposure hierarchy* is often used to plan exposure practices. This tool is discussed later in this chapter.

Exposures Should Be Repeated Frequently

Exposures work best if they are practiced frequently and close together. Imagine how difficult it would be to overcome feeling nervous in a new workplace if you went in only once a month. Daily exposures work better than weekly exposures, and weekly exposures work better than monthly exposures. If practical, we recommend that you initially try some sort of exposure practice at least four or five days each week. For example, if you avoid physical exercise for fear of becoming breathless, try twenty or thirty minutes of aerobic exercises almost daily, until it becomes less scary. Once your fear has decreased, you can spread out your exposure practices.

Try to Make Exposures Prolonged

Exposure works best when practices are prolonged. Ideally, it is best to stay in situations until you learn that your feared consequence is not going to happen, or until your discomfort has decreased to a manageable level. Anxiety typically decreases over the course of an exposure practice, so you will learn that you can be in the situation and, after some time, be unafraid. For example, if you are afraid to visit a hospital, practice walking around the hospital for an hour or two, until you feel more comfortable or learn that nothing bad will happen. If a situation is inherently brief (for example, testing your blood pressure), try repeating the practice over and over, until it is no longer frightening (though, of course, this won't be practical for every possible practice, for example, having a surgical procedure).

Accept Uncomfortable Feelings Rather Than Trying to Control Them

The more you fight your anxiety and fear, the longer you will keep it alive. Instead of trying to control your emotions and physical sensations, the best thing to do is to simply let them happen. Learning to accept your uncomfortable feelings will eventually help to reduce your anxiety and fear.

Eliminate Safety Behaviors

As discussed earlier in this chapter, it is best to eliminate the use of safety behaviors from the start of your treatment. However, if your fear during exposure practices is overwhelming, you can initially include small safety behaviors to help keep your fear at a manageable level during early practices. For example, you might decide to carry a cell phone for the first few practices of a new exposure, such as jogging around the block, if you are anxious about the possibility of an emergency. However, over time, it is useful to decrease your use of safety behaviors.

Confronting Feared Situations

Earlier in this chapter, you generated a list of situations that you fear and avoid. Now is the time to start confronting these situations. Remember, the idea is to do the things that frighten you. So, if your tendency is to visit your doctor *too frequently*, we would recommend decreasing the frequency of your medical visits. On the other hand, if you avoid visiting your doctor because of your anxiety, then we might recommend increasing the frequency of your medical visits until you are no longer afraid. As reviewed earlier, it is important to schedule practices that are predictable, under your control, frequent, and prolonged, if possible. Although you don't need to start with practices that are at the top of your exposure hierarchy, you also don't need to start with practices that are too easy. Ideally practices should be those that are as difficult as you can manage without escaping from the situation.

Exercise: Developing an Exposure Hierarchy

A useful tool for planning your practices is the exposure hierarchy, which is essentially a list of feared situations arranged from the least difficult (at the bottom) to the most difficult (at the top). To develop your own hierarchy, begin with the list you generated earlier of the situations you avoid. Now review your list to see which items might work well on your hierarchy. Ideally, items on your hierarchy should be activities that are practical and possible to arrange. For example, observing open-heart surgery in an operating room might be difficult to arrange; however, more practical items might include watching a video of a surgery online or sitting in the waiting room of a hospital emergency room. Items on your hierarchy should also be as specific as possible, describing the situation in detail. For example, "Go to a hospital" is not as useful an item as "Go to Mount Sinai Hospital and sit in the waiting room of the cancer clinic for an hour."

Typically, exposure hierarchies include ten to fifteen items. If you don't have enough items, you can split some items into more than one. For example, if whether you are alone or accompanied affects your fear, the example item described in the previous paragraph could be split into two items: (1) "Go to Mount Sinai Hospital and sit in the waiting room of the cancer clinic for an hour *with my wife*," and (2) "Go to Mount Sinai Hospital and sit in the waiting room of the cancer clinic for an hour, *alone*." Once you have your list of items, rate your level of fear for each item, using a scale ranging from 0 (no fear at all) to 100 (as frightened as you can imagine being). Then, type up your list in order of difficulty, including your fear estimates. The most difficult items should be at the top, and your list should include items with a wide range of difficulty levels (including items that are moderately anxiety provoking, as well as easier and more difficult items). Once you have developed your hierarchy, you can start to practice the items on your list. Next is an example of an exposure hierarchy.

Sample Exposure Hierarchy		
No.	Situation	Fear (0–100)
1	Visit my family doctor for a checkup, including blood tests.	100
2	Sit in the waiting room of the cancer clinic down the street from me for an hour or until I feel more comfortable (alone).	100
3	Read a book about dying from cancer.	90
4	Sit in the waiting room of the cancer clinic down the street from me for an hour or until I feel more comfortable (with my sister).	85
5	Talk about my uncle's cancer diagnosis with my coworkers.	70
6	Sit in my family doctor's waiting room for an hour alone.	65
7	Test my own blood pressure.	55
8	Watch reruns of "ER" on DVD.	50
9	Sit in my family doctor's waiting room for an hour with my sister.	40
10	Skim an issue of the New England Journal of Medicine.	40

Exercise: Situational Exposure

Now that you have developed an exposure hierarchy, you can begin to practice confronting the situations you fear. Start with items that are more manageable and work up to more-difficult items. Note that you don't need to start at the bottom of your hierarchy. If you feel ready to start with more-difficult items, that's fine. Move on to the next item when your anxiety has decreased to a manageable level, or when you feel ready to try something more difficult. We recommend scheduling practices on at least four or five days a week. If you can practice more frequently, especially in the first few weeks, you will notice improvements more quickly.

After each exposure practice, record in your journal:

1. The date and time of the practice

2. What practice you completed

3. How long you spent on the practice

4. Your maximum level of fear during the practice, using a scale ranging from 0 (no fear) to 100 (as frightened as you can imagine being)

5. How long it took for your fear level to decrease by half

Sample Exposure Log				
Date/ Time	Exposure Task	Minutes Spent	Maximum Fear (0–100)	Minutes to Decrease by Half
July 23/ 2:00 p.m.	Review American Heart Association website	90	90/100	75

Confronting Feared Sensations

Just as confronting feared places, objects, or situations can lead to a reduction in fear of these stimuli, purposely bringing on feared physical symptoms can help to reduce your fear of these sensations. If you are not fearful of physical symptoms, then symptom exposure is not relevant for you. On the other hand, if sensations such as dizziness, racing heart, and breathlessness are frightening to you, then you may find symptom exposure useful. The following table provides examples of exercises you can use to bring on feared sensations, as well as the symptoms they are most likely to trigger.

Symptom Exposure Exercises	
Symptom Exposure Exercise	**Common Sensations Triggered**
Shake your head from side to side (30 sec.)	dizziness, light-headedness
Spin in a swivel chair (60 sec.)	dizziness, light-headedness, unreality, nausea
Hold your breath (30 sec. or for as long as you can)	breathlessness, racing or pounding heart, dizziness, chest tightness
Hyperventilate (breathe quickly, at a rate of about 100–120 breaths per min.) (60 sec.)	breathlessness, dizziness, racing or pounding heart, feeling unreal, trembling or shaking, numbness or tingling sensations
Breathe through a small, narrow straw (plug your nose if necessary, so you aren't tempted to breathe through it) (2 min.)	breathlessness, racing or pounding heart, choking feelings, dizziness, chest tightness, trembling or shaking
Run in place (or up and down stairs) (60 sec.)	racing or pounding heart, breathlessness, chest tightness, sweating, trembling or shaking, blushing

As with situational exposure, you should start with exercises that are less anxiety provoking and work up to more-difficult ones. In addition to these exercises that target specific symptoms, it may also be helpful to practice exposure to any activities or situations you avoid because they trigger sensations you fear. These may include exercise or sports, hot and stuffy rooms, emotional movies, sex, or caffeine, for example.

Exercise: Symptom Exposure

This exercise is relevant only if you are frightened by certain physical sensations. In your journal, make a list of any sensations that make you anxious. Now try the different exercises listed earlier to see which ones bring on your feared symptoms. Skip any exercises for which there is a medical reason you shouldn't do it (check with your doctor if you are not sure). For example, if you have neck pain, skip the exercise that involves shaking your head from side to side. Or if you have asthma or a cold, skip the hyperventilation exercise. For each exercise, record:

1. The date and time

2. What exercise you completed

3. Any sensations triggered by the exercise

4. The level of fear triggered by the exercise, using a scale ranging from 0 (no fear) to 100 (as frightened as you can imagine being)

You can also add more exercises to the list. Can you think of other tasks to bring on the sensations you fear? For example, if feeling hot makes you anxious, you could practice being outside on a hot day, sleeping under warm blankets, sitting in a sauna, drinking a hot drink, wearing warm clothes, or sitting in a hot car.

If you discover that some of these exercises do in fact trigger anxiety or fear, the next step is to practice them repeatedly until they get easier. For example, if hyperventilation makes you anxious, try hyperventilating for sixty seconds. Then take a break for a few minutes until your symptoms subside, and then hyperventilate again. Repeat the exercise six to eight times or until you can experience the physical sensations without much fear. We are not saying that you will experience these sensations without discomfort—no one likes to be dizzy, for example. However, with practice, the discomfort won't be associated with the usual associated fear. We recommend that you practice symptom exposure daily for a few weeks, until the exercises get easier.

Confronting Feared Thoughts and Imagery

Are certain types of thoughts or images frightening to you? If so, exposure to these thoughts and images may lead to decreased anxiety. As reviewed earlier, suppression of anxiety-provoking thoughts often leads to increased distress and frequency of the thoughts. Instead of trying to control your unwanted thoughts, we encourage you to experience them fully. Exposure to frightening thoughts has been shown to reduce anxiety over these thoughts across a number of anxiety problems. Although researchers have not studied the effects of "mental exposure" in people with health anxiety, there is every reason to think that the same processes underlying fear reduction in other anxiety-based problems are relevant in health anxiety as well.

The first step is to identify the thoughts and images that frighten you. Examples might include mental images of yourself in a hospital bed or the thought that you are having a heart attack. Focus on thoughts or images that you tend to interpret as dangerous. If you are generally not frightened of your thoughts, then you can skip this section. However, if you have identified thoughts or images that are threatening to you, the next step is to expose yourself to these mental experiences. You can do this in a number of ways:

Describe the image or thought in writing. Make sure the narrative is detailed and describes the experience using all senses (for example, *seeing* yourself in a hospital bed, *hearing* the sounds of the equipment and the medical staff talking, *feeling* the cold air in the room and your racing heart, *smelling* the familiar "hospital" smell, and so on). Now practice writing it out again and again, until it becomes less frightening.

Describe the feared thought or image aloud. Begin by writing out a detailed script of your feared image or thought (see previous item). Next, read it out loud over and over again, until it is no longer scary.

Have someone else describe your feared image or thought aloud. Begin by writing out a detailed script of your feared image or thought. Next, ask someone else (for example, a close friend, your partner, or a relative) to read your script aloud until hearing it no longer arouses fear.

Record a description of the thought or image. Begin by writing out a description of your feared thought or image. Now, using a computer or another form of technology, read the feared thought or image out loud and record it. Next, listen to your recording repeatedly until it no longer frightens you.

Exercise: Mental Exposure

If you were able to identify thoughts or images that frighten you, plan exposure practices involving repeated exposure to these mental experiences using one or more of the methods described in the previous section. Mental exposure sessions should last twenty to forty minutes, or until the thoughts or images are no longer frightening. We recommend repeating these practices daily for three or four weeks, or until your fear has decreased. In your journal, record:

1. The date and time of each practice

2. A description of the practice

3. Your maximum anxiety or fear during the practice, using a scale from 0 (no anxiety or fear) to 100 (as frightened as you can imagine being)

4. The number of minutes it took for your anxiety or fear to decrease by about half

Exposure and Response Prevention: A Case Example

Manny was a fifty-two-year-old lawyer whose anxiety about his health had been a problem for about five years, ever since his mother had died of pancreatic cancer and his father had suffered a heart attack about three months later. He eventually sought therapy for health anxiety that he described as "nearly constant." His biggest worry was that he might contract cancer, but he also worried about the health of his wife and three children, aged eighteen, twenty-one, and twenty-seven. Whenever he experienced an unusual symptom (including headaches, dizziness, rashes, abdominal pain, skin blemishes, and various other symptoms), he was convinced he had cancer. He had five or six doctors and typically sought reassurance from at least one of them each week.

His worry about the health of his family had begun to affect his relationship with his wife and children. He frequently asked them about their symptoms and, on a regular basis, insisted that they seek medical attention for their own symptoms. For example, when his wife had a pain in her foot for a few days, she and Manny had an argument in which he insisted that she see their family doctor, though she preferred to wait to see whether the pain improved on its own. His constant concern about his family had even led his children to cut back the frequency of their family visits. Although Manny reported using a wide range of safety behaviors (for example, visiting his doctor, asking for reassurance from his family, checking his symptoms and those of his wife and children, reading medical texts, searching for medical information online), he reported that there were no situations that he avoided as a result of his anxiety.

Manny's therapy began with a discussion of the nature of health anxiety and factors that contribute to it, including much of the material that appears in chapter 1 of this book. Next, he spent three weeks monitoring and challenging his anxious thoughts, using the techniques discussed in chapter 3. Using these techniques, Manny came to realize that his anxious beliefs typically did not come true, and he was beginning to see his anxiety as both excessive and unrealistic.

Next, Manny began to use the behavioral strategies described in this chapter. He did not generally avoid situations as a result of his anxiety, so the focus of Manny's treatment was on reducing his use of safety behaviors.

Because Manny's family was very involved in his anxious behaviors, they all joined him for one session of therapy. During this meeting, Manny's wife and children learned the importance of not providing reassurance regarding Manny's symptoms. They learned how, instead, they could provide him with support and encouragement without feeding his need for reassurance about his health. Manny was also instructed not to ask his family for reassurance and not to ask them to see doctors about their own symptoms. He acknowledged that they were all adults and could make their own health care decisions.

Manny also agreed to cut out all health-related Internet searches, reviews of medical books, and visits to his doctor, with the exception of his annual checkup and any additional visits his doctor recommended. Manny was worried that there might be some symptoms that were a sign of some-thing serious, so he reserved the right to visit his doctor no more than once every three months if he experienced a symptom that was unusual or particularly uncomfortable, or that didn't get better after a few weeks.

For the first week, Manny's anxiety became more intense. His urges to check symptoms and ask for reassurance were very strong, and his health worries were interfering with his sleep. On a few occasions, he asked his wife for reassurance about whether particular symptoms might be serious. She just hugged him, told him that she loved him, and reminded him of his therapist's instructions not to provide him with reassurance about his health. Over the next two months, Manny began to see an improvement in his anxiety. He noticed that each time he experienced a scary symptom, it went away on its own, usually within a few hours or days. He continued to experience health anxiety on most days, but it was less intense than it had been before. About once a week, his anxiety became strong, and he used one of his safety behaviors (typically checking the Internet, since he had given up asking his family for reassurance). However, this was much less frequent than it had been in the past, and Manny was pleased with his progress. His family was delighted as well. Manny continued his therapy for a total of five months and continued to make gains even after his therapy ended.

Troubleshooting

This section includes solutions to a few common challenges that often arise when using the behavioral strategies described in this chapter.

Problem:	*My fear does not decrease during my exposure practices.*
Solution:	This can occur for a number of reasons, including you are experiencing high levels of stress in your life, your exposure practice is not predictable or under your control, you are using safety behaviors during your practice, you haven't stayed in the situation long enough to experience a reduction in fear, or you are experiencing negative thinking that undermines the effectiveness of your exposure. If any of these factors seems to be getting in the way of fear reduction for you, deal with it accordingly. For example, try the exposure on a day when you are experiencing less stress, make sure your practice is predictable and under your control, reduce your use of safety behaviors, make sure you stay in the situation long enough, and challenge your negative thinking using the strategies in chapter 3. If all else fails, just keep practicing. Even if your fear doesn't decrease during a particular practice, it will likely decrease between practices, especially if you schedule your exposures close together.
Problem:	*My fear returns between exposure practices.*
Solutions:	Some return of fear between exposure practices is common. In most cases, the amount of fear that returns between exposures is limited, and the less often fear returns, the more practices you complete. Return of fear is often greatest when there is too much time between practices. If you find that most of your fear is returning between practices, try decreasing the time between your exposures. Generally, as discussed earlier in this chapter, we recommend practicing exposure at least four or five times a week.

Problem:	*My fear is too high to benefit from exposure.*
Solution:	We recommend that you choose practices that arouse a fear level of 70 to 80 out of 100, although it is also fine if your fear is a bit higher than that. If you find that your fear is so high that it feels overwhelming or if you are unable to stay in the situation, consider selecting an easier practice from your hierarchy or altering your practice to make it more manageable. These options are preferable to giving up completely. You can also use the strategies from chapter 3 to challenge any anxious thoughts that arise during your exposure practice. If your fear is so strong that you must leave the situation, take a short break and then return to the situation as soon as possible. It's best to end your practice on a good note, once you have achieved some degree of success.

In Brief...

Changing the behaviors that maintain your health anxiety is an important step toward decreasing your fear. Strategies that you use to reduce your anxiety in the short term, such as relying on safety behaviors and avoiding feared situations, feelings, and thoughts, can increase or maintain anxiety over the long term. So it is important to reduce your reliance on these strategies. Instead of avoiding them, confront feared situations directly. Accept feelings of anxiety and fear, rather than try to control them. With practice, your anxiety about your health will improve.

Chapter 5

The Effect of Health Anxiety on Your Relationships

In this chapter we discuss the effects health anxiety often has on relationships. You will be asked to think about your own relationships and to formulate a plan to decrease the impact of health anxiety. If you share this chapter with family and friends, they will also learn skills for decreasing their role in maintaining your health anxiety.

Family and Friends

Annoyance, frustration, and sometimes even anger from people with health anxiety and those who care about them are pretty normal responses. Let's look at why. At first, health fears can seem to strengthen relationships; others in your life may express concern and empathy when they see that you're worried about your health. Health concerns of a family member or friend are often seen as a common enemy; everyone involved has the common goal of wanting the person to be healthy. This mind-set and focus would be helpful and important if you were fighting a serious illness, such as cancer, or recovering from a major surgery. However, if your health anxiety is frequent and out of proportion to any real threat, you have likely found that over time, others have begun to view your health concerns differently than you do. For example, others may have begun to assume that your symptoms are not due to the causes you fear.

This can leave the other people in your life in a difficult situation. On one hand, they really do want you to feel healthy, safe, and secure. On the other hand, others often run out of energy and empathy long before you stop needing it. Constant talk about health anxiety can be very draining on a relationship. Health anxiety may leave you with less to give to your relationships in terms of attention, the ability to do things with others, and the ability to fully consider others. Your partner, family members, and friends can be supportive—driving you to appointments, picking up medications, checking symptoms, missing their own work, worrying, providing reassurance, listening repeatedly to the same list of fears, and so forth—for only so long. At some point, they may expect you to either just "be sick" or "get over it."

Exercise: How Has Your Health Anxiety Affected Your Relationships?

Take a few moments to ask yourself how health anxiety has affected your most important relationships. Examples may include changes for the better (for example, becoming closer) or for the worse (such as spending less time together). After you have listed all the effects you can think of, ask others in your life whether they can think of two or three ways in which they have noticed their relationship with you change. Were there any surprises? Have there been any changes for the better as you have begun to work through this book?

The Reassurance Trap

People who are anxious about their health often feel reassured briefly by health-related information that suggests they may be okay. But, over minutes or hours, the same old doubts and fears tend to creep back into awareness, leaving you feeling no better than before. You may begin to wonder if you heard the doctor incorrectly or if you forgot to describe an important symptom. These types of thoughts can lead to the worry that your diagnosis could be mistaken or incomplete. Anxiety-provoking thoughts and fears can make unlikely possibilities seem likely.

Victoria, for example, had a particularly difficult time with reassurance. Although she asked for people's thoughts, feedback, opinions, and reassurance many times a day, after a few minutes, her own thoughts always turned bleak. She thought maybe her husband and others were offering false reassurance just so she would stop asking. After getting home from the doctor's office, she would begin to focus on how unreliable medical tests can be; they are never 100 percent accurate. If Victoria's doctor referred her for additional tests, she felt better for a while, until her mind stumbled on the idea that if he was ordering tests, he must be worried (versus the much more likely scenario that she had badgered him until he ordered tests he didn't believe were necessary). Once her anxiety reached an uncomfortable level, this cycle would repeat itself and Victoria found herself calling the doctor or asking her husband what he thought—again. This repeated reassurance seeking quickly became counterproductive.

Exercise: Tracking Your Reassurance Needs

Many people with health anxiety underestimate how often they seek reassurance from others. For the next week, pay attention to your own reassurance seeking. Log all instances, no matter how subtle. The tendency to seek reassurance may be routine or a habit for you, and at first you may need others, such as your partner or a friend to point out examples.

In your journal, create a log to include the date and time, the reassurance you asked for, who was involved, the thoughts that led you to look for reassurance, how effective the reassurance was in controlling the anxiety, and (if you feel comfortable asking) how the other person felt when you asked for reassurance. To determine how helpful reassurance is over a longer period of time, rate the effectiveness column twice (as in Mario's example, which follows), once immediately after you are reassured and again the next day or the next time you start feeling the need to seek the same assurances.

Date/ Time	Reassurance Needed	Source of Reassurance	Anxious Thought	Percent Effective in Alleviating Anxiety	How the Other Person Felt
Feb. 18/ 9:02 a.m.	Needed to know that my urine is per-fectly clear, not cloudy at all	Wife	My urine looked like it might be cloudy; I may have a kidney or bladder infection.	75 percent (30 percent next day)	Angry Frustrated Sad

The examples you work on in this exercise can serve as starting points for your daily thought records; you have already pinpointed an anxious thought in each instance. Of course, it is possible that you will have already stopped asking for reassurance, based on the strategies you learned in chapter 4. If that is the case, you can skip over this exercise.

Relief Never Lasts

Reassurance bears a striking similarity to other "quick fixes." By this we mean behaviors that offer relief immediately afterward, such as using alcohol or drugs, shopping excessively, gambling, having sex, yelling, or even giving in to aggressive impulses (like cutting off a slow driver). The urge to engage in these behaviors can feel all-encompassing, overwhelming, and very difficult to delay or resist. Once we give in (for example, by calling the doctor in the example of health anxiety, going to the casino for a gambler, or lighting up for a smoker), the sense of relief is nearly immediate. That feeling—fast relief—can be addictive.

Look at Maggie's example. She found herself increasingly worried that the sore, dry scab by her nostril was getting bigger. She asked her husband, Fred, to look at it carefully each day, wondering aloud if it was bigger than it had been the day before and if it was bigger than it was last week. When she asked Fred, "Do you think it might be skin cancer?" his answer was consistently, "No." As one might expect, no was not enough after a while, and Fred found himself having to explain that he was almost positive; sometimes he would point out, "It's dry skin, just like last winter, from wiping it with tissue all the time." Maggie felt better, but not for very long; she asked the same questions the next day and the next. Like the effects of drugs, alcohol, smoking, and shopping, the effects of reassurance seeking are short lived.

The Role of Reassurance in Maintaining Health Anxiety

As discussed in chapter 4, not only is reassurance short lived, but like other "addictive" behaviors, reassurance seeking perpetuates the problem in the long run. Let's look at another potentially addictive behavior: using alcohol to manage stress or to deal with the desire to drink. Most people will agree that:

🔲 The relief that comes from drinking for these types of reasons is time limited (the person will likely have to drink again in the future).

🔲 Over time, the more alcohol a person drinks, the more that person will need to drink to get the same effect.

🔲 Drinking can perpetuate more drinking; over time people come to believe that they can't handle various situations or stressors without alcohol.

These same principles are true when we consider reassurance seeking and health anxiety:

🔲 The effects of reassurance are time limited, lasting for moments in some cases (for example, when you ask for reassurance many times a day) or longer in other cases (for example, when you visit the doctor every few weeks).

▣ Over time you may require more certainty, evidence, or convincing to experience the same level of relief that you had in the past (you may remember a time when your doctor said that a bit of dizziness was nothing to be concerned about, and you could leave it at that).

▣ Reassurance seeking perpetuates health anxiety by fostering the belief that you will not be able to feel okay, to cope with your anxiety or discomfort, or to cope with not knowing unless you get more reassurance.

Ongoing comforting by family, friends, and doctors ends up leaving you with more doubt and discomfort, rather than less. Excessive reassurance seeking makes you less able to believe your own logical reasoning (something you are working on with your daily thought records), and leads to increased anxiety and more of those anxiety-related symptoms you identified in chapter 1.

Exercise: Decreasing Your Need for Reassurance

Using a log like the situational exposure one in chapter 4, track an instance of purposefully *not* asking for reassurance. Although the urge to be reassured may increase initially, your discomfort and desire for reassurance should decrease over time. As you complete this exercise, don't give in to the desire to alleviate your anxiety immediately with reassurance. Instead, track your level of discomfort and see how long the desire to seek reassurance remains at its peak level. Continue the exposure until the anxiety decreases somewhat or until you learn that your feared consequence doesn't come true. As you continue your daily exposure and response-prevention exercises, include instances like this one. Expose yourself to situations in which the desire to seek reassurance, information, or a second opinion is strong, and then face up to your anxiety: do the opposite of what you usually do and watch the anxiety lessen over time, with each repetition. An added benefit of this type of exercise will be gradual improvements in any relationships that are strained by repeated requests for reassurance.

Mario, for example, recorded many instances in which he experienced a strong fear that his cloudy urine was a sign of some terrible illness. When completing this exercise, he entered the following item at the top of his exposure log: "Urinate without asking my wife to examine for cloudiness." Mario did just that. He urinated as usual and left it in the bowl to really put his willpower to the test; he felt a strong desire to ask his wife the typical string of questions. Partly, asking had become a habit, but the main reason for asking was a rising level of anxiety and uncertainty. Mario felt that he couldn't trust his own judgment and that all of the other times his wife had assured him that nothing was wrong somehow didn't count. He felt that this time was different; he always felt that *this* situation was different. Despite that feeling, Mario chose not to ask his wife to check his urine.

Initially, Mario's anxiety reached a level of 80 out of 100. He was surprised to find that over the course of ninety minutes (without distraction), his anxiety, discomfort, and the feeling that he needed his wife's reassurance had decreased to a manageable 30 out of 100. After repeating this task several times a day for a week, Mario realized that he could completely stop asking his wife to take part in this process, which both of them had found embarrassing. Not only can family relationships be improved as Mario's did, but so can your relationship with your doctor.

You and Your Doctor

The following practical guidelines regarding your relationship with your doctor, when to see the doctor, and how to make the most of medical appointments will not only improve relations with health care providers, but also help your health anxiety decrease in the long run.

Good relationships are characterized by meaningful and respectful communications, mutual understanding, openness, trust, and confidence. If you have a good relationship with your doctor, you will be more likely to receive timely service and appropriate action. When we experience responsive care and believe we are being well cared for, most of us can more readily accept the conclusions and opinions of our physicians.

Kathleen, for example, experienced a very long period when she was inexplicably nauseated. Weeks and months went by with her feeling unwell most days until about lunchtime. Her doctor was diligent, completing the requisite blood tests, checking for pregnancy, ulcers, and viruses. He prescribed a strong antacid for Kathleen that did not prove useful. After a number of appointments, the doctor was of the opinion that Kathleen's stomach problems were most likely owing to stress. After this appointment, Kathleen began to consider the possibility that thinking about being nauseous and constantly monitoring how her stomach felt, what she was eating, and if she could easily leave situations were contributing to her nausea. Although she continued to worry off and on about whether something had been missed, Kathleen took her doctor's assertion to heart. Although the problem took several months to resolve completely, nothing serious ever came of her symptoms.

Unfortunately many people with health anxiety report that over time, their doctor-patient relationships deteriorate. At first, you may experience feeling generally unheard or perhaps as though your concerns are not being taken seriously enough. You may begin to wonder if your doctor is staying up to date or is beginning to become obsolete or jaded. These types of complaints are quite common in people with elevated health anxiety, and when the trust and respect in such a relationship begins to decline, health anxiety may increase.

Think back to the example of Kathleen's nausea. Had her relationship with Dr. Joseph been weaker, she would have found it more difficult to accept his judgment and nearly impossible to stop looking for explanations. Her doctor could have easily taken a misstep by seeing her less frequently (leading Kathleen to worry that she wasn't being taken seriously) or continuing to order test after test (and feeding into her fear that some serious problem was yet to be discovered). Either of these responses may have set the stage for worsening health anxiety. For her part, Kathleen could have been more demanding or less willing to trust her doctor's opinion (jeopardizing the relationship and making herself less able to believe in him). This, too, would have set the stage for the development of even greater health anxiety.

Or Kathleen could have avoided her physician completely. The outcome would likely have been increased tension, worry, and fear. Many people believe that those with anxiety about their health spend too much time at doctors' offices and that they invariably use more than their share of medical resources. While this can be true, some people with health anxiety do everything they can to avoid medical care, in the same way that others with health anxiety may avoid television programs about disease or ill people. This can also present a problem, and as such, balance is an important goal.

In instances where the doctor-patient relationship is severely stressed, a physician may stop seeing a patient completely, or patients may begin looking for alternative opinions. Occasionally seeking a second opinion, especially if your doctor suggests it, can be a useful and adaptive endeavor. On the other hand, overreliance on doctor shopping will contribute to health anxiety.

Doctor Shopping

Repeatedly changing doctors, seeing more than one doctor simultaneously, or consistently seeking second, third, and fourth opinions can be very tempting. Under normal circumstances, if you believe that you're not receiving adequate service (from your doctor, lawyer, waiter, or child's teacher), you might be encouraged to do something about it. You might take action by making a comment, complaining to management, or leaving that service provider for another. Normally you might benefit from improved service this way. But doctor shopping, like reassurance seeking or symptom monitoring, works against those with health anxiety.

A solid relationship with your physician is built over time. Trust often builds slowly, and you can't necessarily expect to feel complete trust for your physician immediately. Many of the exercises you have completed in this book already involve testing a prediction that you aren't sure of (for example, that your anxiety will decrease even if you don't check your heart rate). By repeating these experiments on a regular basis, you can slowly begin to trust that these hypotheses are often true and that your feared outcome typically never happens. In the same way, it is important to tentatively accept your physician's opinion, wait, and then find out what happens. Over many repetitions, it becomes much easier to accept what your doctor suggests; you will have lots of evidence from the past. This does not happen if you are doctor shopping. When doctor shopping, you don't get the repeated experience of accepting your doctor's opinion and discovering that it is typically valid. Doctor shopping also leads to unnecessary tests and appointments, because a new physician has to bring herself up to speed on your health.

The Other Side of the Desk

If you believe that your doctor doesn't give you answers that are absolute, definitive, bulletproof, unambiguous, or beyond question, that's because you're right. Many health care providers (not just physicians) tend to avoid definitive statements. When you or I ask a doctor for definitive information about a diagnosis or condition (for example, "Are you positive? Are you sure I don't have lupus? Are you sure that this isn't early dementia?"), there's a good chance that the response will come with a qualifier. Frequently used qualifiers may include:

- "I can't say for 100 percent sure, but,…"

- "What this looks like to me is…"

- "It is highly unlikely that…"

- "There are no guarantees, but…"

- "Although no test is foolproof…"

- "Ninety-nine percent of the time…"

- "Feel free to get a second opinion, but…"

For people without health anxiety, this type of response is expected and is loosely interpreted to mean, "Yes, I *am* sure, but I can't say I'm perfectly sure because of the one in a million chance that I might be wrong." Unfortunately, people with health anxiety often don't benefit from these qualified assurances, which may be aimed at avoiding being sued for malpractice. People with health anxiety prefer information spoken with surety, yet this is just not how most health care providers speak. It does not mean they aren't confident, nor does it mean that they doubt their findings, are secretly worried about you, or are hiding something.

It can be extremely frustrating for physicians to work with patients they believe they are not helping, and often this is the case for patients with high levels of health anxiety. If you are very anxious about your health, and feel that something is seriously wrong and that you are not being helped, you may feel irritable, scared, or helpless. You may call or go to your doctor's office more often than most patients, and may leave feeling no better.

From the other side of the doctor's desk, patients with health anxiety may seem demanding, angry, needy, and upset. Of course, most people would be angry, needy, or upset if they had anxious beliefs about their health, but this can be frustrating for your doctor. Nothing she does seems to help; in fact the situation often gets worse with time. Little that the doctor says is believed. Imagine for a moment what it might be like if you had an employer, a colleague, or an acquaintance asking for your help or expertise. At first you would probably be glad to help in whatever way you felt was right and appropriate—after all, you're the expert. Now imagine what it would be like if the person consistently second-guessed your conclusions; ignored your advice; went for a second opinion; or asked you the same question a week later, two weeks later, and three weeks later. How many times would this have to happen before you became frustrated? How many times has this cycle taken place between you and your doctor?

In the same way that frequent symptom checking, avoiding situations, and seeking reassurance from family can be mitigated by carrying out gradual exposure tasks, so can doctor shopping and other relationship-sabotaging behaviors. These behaviors include visiting the doctor's office or hospital too often, calling too frequently, arriving at the doctor's office with a long list of symptoms and concerns each time, treating your doctor or his staff disrespectfully, focusing on a complaint that your doctor has told you does not need further attention, arriving at your appointments armed with Internet information questioning your doctor's judgment, and insisting that your doctor agree with your self-diagnosis. In all likelihood, no matter how lax, careless, or rushed you think your doctor is, unless you also have a medical degree, your doctor is probably more skilled at the process of diagnosis and treatment at her worst than you would be at your best.

Exercise: Exposure, Again

Start a new sheet in your journal. This entry will be an exposure task, like those you have been working on from chapter 4. This exposure, however, should be designed to bring on anxiety that you typically deal with by interacting with a medical professional. Remember, exposure is always meant to make you feel moderately anxious, and then have you cope with that feeling. Rate your anxiety before, during, and after your exposure task. Some examples include:

- Delay visiting your physician for a symptom you have already had cleared.

- Delay calling your doctor, nurse, or health line.

- Once you have received information or advice from your doctor, choose not to seek a second opinion.

As with your previous exposure exercises, decide on your task and then track your level of discomfort using a rating from 0 (no anxiety or discomfort) to 100 (as anxious or uncomfortable as you can imagine being), and see how long the anxiety remains at its peak level. Continue the exposure until the anxiety has decreased somewhat, or long enough to learn that your feared consequence doesn't come true. As you continue your daily exposure exercises, include instances like this one. Expose yourself to situations that typically make you want to see your doctor and then act in the face of anxiety: do the opposite of what you usually do and watch your discomfort lessen with time and with each repetition.

Seeing Your Doctor

Of course, even people who are anxious about their health are sometimes sick or injured, or need medication, tests, or treatment. Therefore, there will be times when you ought to see your doctor. If you are used to going to your doctor more often than the typical healthy person who isn't anxious about his health (more than once or twice a year), it may be helpful to develop some guidelines to help you decide whether to visit your doctor in any particular situation. Setting an appointment with your doctor to work together at developing a list of situations when you should seek medical care can go a long way toward improving the relationship, educating your physician about health anxiety, and demonstrating your commitment to change—even when it is difficult. The material in this section builds on the discussion in chapter 4 on how to decide whether to seek medical attention.

Scheduling Regular Visits

Scheduling regular visits with your physician (regardless of whether you feel well or unwell) is important for several reasons. This type of appointment scheduling breaks the pattern of visiting the doctor because you feel anxious, receiving reassurance, and then experiencing a brief drop in anxiety (which, as you remember, can be like an addiction). Regularly scheduled appointments also allow your physician to check in on your health-anxiety progress and to monitor any existing health conditions, such as high blood pressure or obesity.

Exercise: Working Together

Make an appointment with your doctor to discuss and agree on a schedule of regular appointments and additional situations in which a visit would be called for. Check off the situations that you both agree are reasonable.

- ☐ Yearly physical

- ☐ Scheduled visits every _____ weeks (for example, every eight or ten weeks might be appropriate if you have a condition that requires monitoring)

- ☐ To receive a prescription renewal

- ☐ To receive vaccinations (for example, for seasonal influenza)

☐ If you experience a significant change to a preexisting condition. List your conditions here: _____

_____

_____

If you develop new symptoms, such as a cough or fever, that last for a period you and your doctor agree on (specify period here): _____

Getting the Most Out of Your Appointments

Many people, not just those with health anxiety, often feel as though they don't know how to handle doctors' appointments. Most of us occasionally believe we haven't communicated our concerns clearly, don't exactly remember what the doctor said, or think of something important half an hour after the meeting has ended. The following tips for maximizing the benefits of your appointments are useful for anyone. They will be especially useful for you as you work toward going to the doctor's office, walk-in clinic, or hospital less frequently. When you do go:

▣ Bring a list of items that are particularly important to have addressed. This does not mean you should bring an extensive, lengthy, detailed log of every one of your symptoms. A reasonable set of items to discuss during a checkup may include questions about your weight, adding your aunt's cancer to your family history, reporting that you are worried because your knuckles have recently been swollen and sore (unless you have already discussed this), and asking for a renewal of your prescriptions. Double-check your list at the end of the appointment to be sure you've mentioned everything.

▣ Bring a list of prescriptions, over-the-counter medications, and supplements you are currently taking, along with dosages and the reason you are taking each.

◙ If you don't understand something, say so. When people are unsure of what someone is saying, it's very easy to assume that the person means something different than she in fact does. In the case of health anxiety, ambiguous health-related information is likely to be interpreted in a negative or frightening way.

◙ Bring some paper (perhaps your health-anxiety journal) to write down important information. Once you have written it down (for example, "The cough is bronchitis; fill the prescription and see the doctor again in two weeks"), ask your doctor to read it over quickly for errors.

Visits to the Emergency Room

When you are extremely frightened about a symptom and believe you are in danger, going to the emergency room may seem like a reasonable and smart option. That said, many people who are anxious about their health have gone to the emergency room (some of them, many times) only to be told that there is nothing seriously wrong or that they should not have come in. Although that may be true—and most of the time people do not need to seek emergency services—we are rarely told under what circumstances we *should* go. This leaves each situation open to interpretation, and when you are highly anxious is not the best time for you to make a decision based on the facts. You are much more likely to make cognitive errors (such as catastrophic thinking) under these kinds of conditions. Therefore, it will be useful for you to know before you are in a health-anxiety-provoking situation when it is appropriate to go to emergency and, by deduction, when it is not.

How do people who aren't particularly worried about their health know when a medical condition rises to the level of a medical emergency? The American College of Emergency Physicians (2010) offers a list of warning signs that indicate a medical emergency. You should go to an emergency department (or call for an ambulance) if you experience:

◙ Difficulty breathing or shortness of breath

- ▣ Chest or upper-abdominal pain or pressure

- ▣ Fainting, sudden dizziness, weakness

- ▣ Changes in vision

- ▣ Confusion or changes in mental status

- ▣ Any sudden or severe pain

- ▣ Uncontrolled bleeding

- ▣ Severe or persistent vomiting or diarrhea

- ▣ Coughing or vomiting of blood

- ▣ Suicidal feelings

- ▣ Difficulty speaking

- ▣ Unusual abdominal pain

Exercise: When to Go to Emergency

The next time you are at your doctor's office, check to see if she has anything to add or remove from the list, above, of reasons to go to the emergency room. It is particularly important to discuss symptoms that, for you, may typically be owing to anxiety. For example, if you typically experience shortness of breath or dizziness when anxious, you would need to watch for shortness of breath or sudden dizziness that feels unusual. Add the information to your journal.

Information for Family and Friends

This section is written primarily for loved ones of people who experience high levels of health anxiety. Family and friends can play an important role in recovery from health anxiety. Health anxiety in the family can lead to disorder, confusion, discord, and hard feelings. In addition to leading to angry and frustrated feelings, family members' efforts to be helpful and supportive may lead to unintentional reinforcement of health anxiety. If you are a family member (or friend) of someone with health anxiety, you may be frustrated not only with your loved one, but with your own responses as well.

Take Graham, for example. When he sat down and thought about it, Graham could not believe how involved he had become in his twenty-eight-year-old daughter's anxiety. He was driving her to appointments almost daily and providing reassurance on the phone at all hours of the day and night. Lately, she had even convinced him to call her employer and explain why she wouldn't be at work. What had happened, he wondered, to his bright, independent daughter? At times he felt as though he were to blame.

It's Normal to Want to Help a Loved One Feel Better

Throughout this book we've emphasized the cyclical nature of health anxiety, and you likely have experienced this as well. At first, it makes perfect sense to provide reassurance, concern, support, and practical help. Depending on the person, this might include going to the emergency room, going on doctors' visits, picking up prescriptions, helping pay medical bills, or taking part in various checking behaviors. What seems reasonable at first, like feeling a mole to see if it is raised, can become complex and nearly ridiculous over time, such as photographing and measuring a mole twice a day.

What Can You Do?

Start by asking the person with health anxiety how he would like you to be involved in this process of self-help. This may involve small changes, like reminding the person to spend some time on the exercises in this book each day, or larger changes, like agreeing to stop taking the person to the emergency room for symptoms that have already been addressed.

One of the unhelpful ways in which friends and family members deal with the disruption and anxiety caused by excessive health fears is to take part in health-anxiety behaviors. Although some of these actions appear helpful at first glance, they serve to reinforce the grip health anxiety has on the thoughts and beliefs of the very person you are trying to help. In the next section we'll offer some positive alternatives. Following is a list of common ways in which family members and friends participate in health anxiety, which are also areas to consider changing:

- Responding with reassuring phrases (for example, "You're okay," "The doctor said it's nothing to worry about," "It looks fine to me," "You're not going to die") every time the person with health anxiety asks about a symptom or fear

- Facilitating or encouraging health-monitoring behaviors (for example, checking blood pressure, pulse, temperature, or other areas of concern)

- Driving the person with health anxiety to unnecessary appointments or otherwise helping that person to seek medical reassurance (for example, calling the doctor or health line)

- Helping to pay for health-related expenses, including tests, procedures, medications, or supplements

- Protecting the person with health anxiety from upsetting situations or information (for example, throwing away the newspaper or changing the television channel if health information comes up)

- Avoiding places or substances that cause the person with health anxiety to become upset

- Trying to reason with the person who has health anxiety—by offering logic, theories, and facts about brain tumors, multiple sclerosis, or heart disease, for example—because as with all reassurance, the effect is likely to be short lived

Planned Disengagement

It would be best to work together to come up with a plan for disengagement before changing your behavior. It would probably cause a great deal of anxiety and disruption if you stopped providing reassurance and taking part in anxiety-related behaviors with your loved one without first discussing it with her. The help of a therapist familiar with the treatment of anxiety problems may be useful at this point. You may also benefit from reading this book in its entirety to better understand what your friend, partner, or family member with health anxiety is working on.

As your friend or loved one works through this book, it is appropriate for you to consider changing your own behaviors. How are you going to gradually stop taking part in activities that reinforce health anxiety? Here are some guidelines that may be useful as you sit down together to chart a course of action:

- Recognize that stress, anger, and frustration in the household are likely to increase your loved one's anxiety and make it more difficult for him to take the necessary steps to change.

- Do your best to manage your own anger and frustration. Don't blame your loved one for his health anxiety.

- Provide support for the positive steps your loved one takes, but don't nag the person to practice more frequently.

- Unless your loved one has given you permission to do so, avoid the temptation to correct his behavior if he slips up (for example, if he asks for reassurance).

- As you reduce the frequency with which you provide reassurance, recognize that your loved one's anxiety may increase initially before it begins to improve.

- Stop providing reassurance and participating in your loved one's anxiety safety behaviors. Before making these changes, however, be sure to discuss this process with your loved one, so she understands why you are changing your behaviors. Explain that although you will no longer support the anxiety, you will continue to be there for your loved one and to support her efforts to overcome the anxiety.

- If completely eliminating your involvement is impossible at first, find ways (in consultation with your loved one) to reduce your involvement gradually (for example, reduce the frequency of providing reassurance, or try adding a delay before providing reassurance).

- Anticipate that your loved one may show some resistance to the changes you are making. It's important to discuss these changes with the person from time to time so that your reasons for making the changes are clear.

- Respond to requests for reassurance in a calm and supportive way, using phrases such as:

  - "If I provide you with reassurance, it will only help to keep your anxiety alive over the long term."

  - "I know that answering that question would make you feel better now, but it won't help over the long run."

  - "Your therapist (or book) told us that if I can resist the temptation to provide you with reassurance, together we can beat this problem."

  - "I know it's difficult, but it's best if I don't call your doctor for you."

Exercise: Disengagement Schedule

Now that you have an idea about what sorts of behavior may be contributing to health anxiety, work together to come up with a schedule for eventual disengagement. The following is an example of the first two weeks in a six-week plan:

Dates	Behavioral Changes for a Family Member of a Person with Health Anxiety
July 14–21	• Stop proofreading the newspaper and hiding articles about cancer. • Stop double-checking the medications.
July 22–29	• Stop providing reassurance about the color of John's tongue. • Begin watching medical dramas together once a week despite discomfort.

Stick with It

You worked on the disengagement schedule together and have likely agreed on most of the items, in principle. That said, when the time actually comes to deny your family member or friend the reassurance or help she wants so badly, it may be difficult to stand firm. It is much easier, especially in the heat of the moment, to give in or say one more time, "Everything is fine," or that you are sure the headache is "nothing serious." It can feel hard-hearted or cruel to refuse to drive to the doctor's office despite pleas that this time something is really wrong. You will always have to use your own judgment and do what you feel is right. That said, giving in to health anxiety keeps it alive and can make it worse in the long run; of that there is no doubt. Standing firm, siding *with* your family member *against* health anxiety, may be difficult, but in the long run you can be part of the solution.

In Brief...

In this chapter you learned more about how health anxiety affects your relationships with family, friends, and health care providers. You also learned how reassurance can perpetuate health anxiety, and you began to consider how you can improve relations with those in your life.

Chapter 6

Strategies for Dealing with Stress

High levels of stress at work, at home, or in other aspects of your life can increase the intensity of negative emotions such as anxiety and depression. Using tools to manage daily stress may help to decrease your level of background arousal, thereby reducing your overall level of anxiety and distress. This chapter provides you with strategies for dealing more effectively with the stresses that arise in your daily life.

The strategies in this chapter are somewhat different from those discussed in previous chapters. Previously, we emphasized the importance of *not* avoiding. We encouraged you to face uncomfortable thoughts, sensations, emotions, and situations, and to accept the anxiety that these experiences bring. When it comes to excessive or unrealistic health-related anxiety, facing your fears is an important part of overcoming them. In this chapter, we discuss strategies for dealing with real stresses: those that most people would agree are stressful (for example, actual health issues, family stresses, long work hours, financial strain, and so on). Here, exposing yourself to more stress is not the answer. Instead, the best approach is to find ways to cope better with stressful situations (for example, learning to relax) and to reduce the amount of life stress you experience on a day-to-day basis (for example, arranging to get help with an excessive workload).

In this chapter, we will focus on three strategies for managing stress: mindfulness-based strategies, breathing retraining, and progressive muscle relaxation. If your life is particularly stressful, check out the latest edition of *The Relaxation and Stress Reduction Workbook* (New Harbinger Publications, 2008).

As we have mentioned throughout this book, avoidance contributes to excessive health anxiety in the long run. Note that there is a very important distinction between using these techniques to manage general day-to-day anxiety, worries, and stress, and using them to avoid the thoughts and physical symptoms that trigger your health anxiety. Using the techniques in this chapter to cope with everyday stresses or to work toward becoming a generally less-anxious person is likely to be useful. Distracting yourself from health anxiety (especially during your health-anxiety-exposure practices) with these strategies is not useful, and may even make your exposure practices less valuable.

Anxiety Management Strategies

We suggest trying each of these skills for at least a few weeks. While you continue working on your daily thought records and exposure tasks, practice these more general strategies once or twice a day (but, again, don't use these techniques to distract yourself from your health anxiety). You can find more information about these techniques in the resources section in the back of this book. The material we present here is really just an introduction. As always, use common sense when you are trying new exercises. If you have reason to believe that any of following techniques may be risky for you (for example, neck pain that worsens when you tighten the muscles of your neck during progressive muscle relaxation), double-check with your doctor at your next scheduled appointment.

Mindfulness

The practice of mindfulness grew out of Zen Buddhism, Western contemplative practices, and Eastern meditation. Mindfulness has been proposed as a useful framework for people with a wide variety of concerns. For example, mindfulness-based strategies can be used effectively to reduce the likelihood of relapse in depression (Williams et al. 2007) and to reduce symptoms of generalized anxiety and worry (Orsillo and Roemer 2011).

What Is Mindfulness?

If you were to look for the definition of mindfulness in a hundred places, you would undoubtedly find a hundred slightly different descriptions. It can be helpful to think of mindfulness as two related processes: being fully engaged in the moment; and purposefully taking a nonjudgmental stance, acknowledging that your thoughts and feelings are just thoughts and feelings. Mindfulness is maximized when we are both fully attentive to the physical realities of the present and aware that our thoughts and emotions are fleeting.

In the Moment

Being fully engaged in the moment means different things to different people. For us, this refers to noticing your current place in the world, noticing your surroundings as filtered through your senses. Your senses are the edge (the border, if you will) where you meet your environment. On one side of the border is the physical world, everything outside yourself, be it people, objects, noises, or fragrances. On the other side of the border is your internal world, everything fully within yourself, such as thoughts, opinions, plans, memories, and feelings. To be fully engaged in the moment, we ask that you direct your focus to the border, that place where each of your senses meets the world. What do you hear, smell, taste, feel, and see right this moment, in your present?

Passing Thoughts and Feelings

All of us have a mental commentator. Sometimes this is referred to as an inner voice or your thought processes. Most of what we are doing in our minds at any given moment tends to be a mishmash of attending to our senses (as discussed earlier) and thinking various thoughts. These thoughts are "the commentator." You might be reviewing the past, making predictions about the future, judging, deciding, assigning value, and so on. At times, the commentator can be so engaging that we find it difficult to be fully in the present. Have you ever read a page and then realized you did not remember a word of it, driven to work without noticing anything that happened along your route, gobbled down a hamburger without tasting it, or asked someone how she was doing without ever hearing her reply? You were probably distracted by thoughts or emotions. Sometimes we believe that our thoughts and emotions are real, objective, or factual, and forget that they are only mental content. You do not need to judge them, label them, push them out of your awareness, fight against them, or always act on them. They will pass.

Being Mindfully Present

Mindfulness does not have to fit into a formal program of meditation, and your acts of mindfulness do not have to look like anyone else's. That said, if the little bit we've been able to include here piques your interest to learn more or to try some of the more-formal mindfulness techniques, there are good resources to choose from. See the resources section.

You can practice simple mindfulness anytime and anywhere. You don't have to lie down, breathe a certain way, meditate, or hold a yoga pose. Being mindful is a matter of realizing what is happening in the present moment and noticing your mind's usual commentary without acting on it.

Walking can become an exercise in mindfulness if you pay attention to your senses: the feel of your feet; the swish of your arms; the breeze touching your hair and drying your eyes; the feel of your breath going in and out of your lungs; the alternating warmth and coolness as you walk from sunny to shady patches; the sound of your steps, your breath, the wind in the grass; and the sights and smells that surround you. Rachelle found that after some practice, walking mindfully became easier. She also found that when she paid close attention to what she was actually experiencing in the world at any given moment, the physical sensations that had so worried her (a headache and sore eyes) became two of many sensations, rather than the only two in her awareness.

As Rachelle practiced walking mindfully, she found that she was often pulled off track by her thoughts—by the commentator. One minute Rachelle would be walking mindfully, and the next she would be thinking that she would have to rush supper if it was to be ready on time. As thoughts often do, the topic jumped from supper to groceries to her daughter's picky eating. Then Rachelle caught herself and thought, *I'm not supposed to be thinking of all this stuff! Now I've goofed up this exercise!* She felt a sense of defeat.

This is precisely where the second facet of mindfulness comes in: accepting your thoughts and feelings just as they are. Rachelle remembered that her thoughts were neither good nor bad, proper nor improper, right nor wrong; they were just thoughts. As though they were leaves floating by in a stream at her feet, Rachelle noticed each thought and emotion with curiosity and interest (for example, *That's cool; my mind wandered from supper to my daughter. I was making a mental grocery list. I felt a sense of defeat*). Then she let these thoughts go by without fighting or judging them. Once you have done this—noticed your thoughts and feelings, and watched them pass—you can gently bring your attention back to your senses. For Rachelle this meant going back to walking mindfully without judging herself for having been briefly distracted. Being distracted isn't inherently positive or negative; it just is. You may use mindfulness to notice thoughts related to health anxiety (such as *I really feel that I should check my blood pressure*) without acting on them.

Exercise: Being Fully in the Moment

One way of building mindfulness into your everyday life is by using cues that will give your attention a nudge (just like putting your vitamins beside your toothbrush to help you remember to take them in the morning). One example of an environmental cue might be opening doors. You might choose to practice being mindful every time you open a door. As you open the door and continue your task (be it walking up the stairs or starting the car), notice your sensations and the situation in which you find yourself. Attend to the feel of the door handle in your hand. Is it warm or cool? Is it smooth or rough? Is it made of metal, plastic, or wood? Does it reflect the light? Is there a sound as you open the door? What are you thinking? Remember, you are simply noticing things—temperature, sound, light, your thoughts about these and other things—and watching the thoughts float past.

If mindfully opening doors doesn't feel quite right for you, choose another cue that fits better. Some examples include picking up a broom or mop as you set about chores, squirting dish soap into the sink, or taking the first bite of a lovely meal—mindfully.

Exercise: Logging Your Mindfulness Practices

Many people find that mindfulness takes some practice. To determine whether mindfulness is a useful skill for you, make a log in your journal. Once a day, record the following information: date and time, mindfulness task, ability to focus on sensations (using a scale from 0, meaning completely unable, to 100, meaning completely able), and ability to let thoughts and emotions pass (again, using a scale from 0 to 100). Here is an example.

Date and Time	Mindfulness Task	Ability to Focus on Sensations	Ability to Let Thoughts and Emotions Pass
July 14/ 7:00 p.m.	Dusting	50	20
July 15/ 7:00 p.m.	Petting the dog	80	65

Breathing Retraining

Research has demonstrated that subtle shifts in breathing can cause anxiety symptoms, including numbness or tingling in the hands, feet, and lips; light-headedness; dizziness; headache; chest pain; and a sense of breathlessness (Barlow 2002).

Hyperventilation

The symptoms listed above are particularly common when people tend to *hyperventilate,* or breathe more quickly or deeply than they need to. Hyperventilation is common when people are under stress, and among people who experience high levels of anxiety. The symptoms caused by incorrect breathing can sometimes lead to unnecessary visits to family doctors and mistaken trips to the emergency room.

The sensation of not getting enough air is a common experience of people who are hyperventilating. In fact, the opposite is true. Hyperventilation (or overbreathing) means that because you are breathing too quickly or too deeply, you expel carbon dioxide (CO_2) faster than your body can produce it. Hyperventilation reduces the CO_2 concentration of your blood to below its normal level, thereby making your blood slightly less acidic. Although harmless, hyperventilation leads to constriction of the blood vessels supplying your brain and extremities, which leads to sensations such as light-headedness and the other sensations described earlier. These changes account for a wide array of symptoms that are virtually identical to the symptoms of anxiety. Even a deep breath or sigh can trigger symptoms in someone who chronically overbreathes. In fact, some people may be symptomatic most of the time. Others are symptomatic only during a stressful period or when they're feeling anxious.

Causes of hyperventilation. Sometimes hyperventilation can be obvious. More often, though, overbreathing occurs more subtly, and you may not even know you are doing it. When stressed or worried, you likely tense the muscles in your neck, throat, chest, and abdomen. This type of muscular tensing (especially in the abdomen) leads to rapid breaths. This type of breathing tends to be centered in the upper chest region and is sometimes called "chest breathing." As the drop in CO_2 causes distressing symptoms, you may become afraid of them. Arousal then remains high, and a cycle of anxiety and anxiety-related sensations occurs.

You may find this next fact interesting: hyperventilation is more likely when you are stressed and immobile or relatively still than when you are moving around. Sitting or lying down is often a natural response to frightening or uncomfortable sensations; unfortunately it tends to make overbreathing (and the symptoms that come with overbreathing) more likely. As an experiment, next time you experience anxiety-related symptoms (refer back to chapter 1 for a list), try some light activity like walking up and down stairs, vacuuming, or walking the dog for a few minutes. See if you notice any difference in how you feel.

How do you know if you hyperventilate? Many people are relieved when they find out that some of their symptoms are due to overbreathing. Here are a few hints that your style of breathing might be contributing to your symptoms:

- ▣ Breathing fourteen or more breaths a minute

- ▣ Breathing mostly from the upper part of the chest (in other words, instead of having your stomach move in and out as in normal breathing, your breastbone, neck, shoulder, or collarbones move)

- ▣ Frequent deep breaths, sighing, or yawning

The effects of overbreathing can be mitigated by changing your breathing style or by increasing the amount of CO_2 produced by your body through physical exercise.

Abdominal Breathing

There are two main muscle groups involved in breathing. The first is the *diaphragm*, which is a sheetlike muscle that runs along the bottom of the rib cage. When the diaphragm contracts, it moves down, expanding the chest cavity and allowing air to flow into the lungs. We exhale when the diaphragm relaxes. Diaphragmatic breathing causes the lower part of the lungs to expand and contract, causing the abdomen to move. The second muscle group involved in breathing, the *intercostal muscles*, are those located between the ribs that allow the rib cage to expand and contract so that air can flow in and out of the lungs. Breathing that relies primarily on the intercostal muscles (chest breathing) causes expansion of the upper part of the lungs and more movement in the chest area.

Normally breathing is slow, effortless, regular, fluid, and quiet, and ideally the diaphragm does most of the work. However, people sometimes overuse their intercostal muscles for breathing, which tends to be a less relaxing way to breathe. Abdominal breathing involves shifting from using primarily the intercostal muscles for breathing to using the diaphragm. Some people are able to master abdominal breathing with little difficulty; others may require considerable practice. The goal is to change from rapid (chest) breathing to slow, regular, rhythmic (abdominal) breathing. After some practice, you may find that this becomes more automatic.

Learning to breathe abdominally can result in positive changes in your physical symptoms and in your anxiety. Here is one technique for learning to breathe more abdominally:

1. Lie on your back or sit in a reclined position. (The first time, you may want to put a pillow under your head so you can watch your stomach.)

2. Loosen tight clothing (belts, ties, collars).

3. Take a few seconds to relax your entire body, especially your stomach muscles, chest, shoulders, neck, face, and jaw.

4. Place a book on your abdomen (right around your navel).

5. Breathe in comfortably and rhythmically (but not deeply), through your nose. As you breathe in, let your stomach rise slowly; the book should gradually rise, as if your stomach were a balloon filling gently with air.

6. Move smoothly into the exhalation with little pause. As you slowly exhale, the book should gently fall, as the "balloon" deflates.

When you breathe with your diaphragm, the abdomen expands when you inhale and contracts when you exhale. If you are able to make the book move up and down, try the exercise without the book, and then try it while sitting up or standing. With practice, you will likely be able to breathe using your diaphragm in just about any position.

Exercise: Correcting Your Breathing

Now that you know what abdominal breathing looks and feels like, it's time for you to try it consistently for a while. Here are some suggested guidelines:

▣ Practice twice a day for five to ten minutes each time (for example, when your clock radio goes off in the morning, practice your breathing throughout two songs before you get up).

▣ For the first few days, just breathe at your regular rate; if at any point you feel dizzy, stop practicing for a while (you might need to build up gradually to five minutes over a few days).

▣ Be sure that you are not breathing too quickly or deeply; just breathe slowly and regularly.

▣ After about a week, begin to gradually slow your breathing rate to about four seconds for each breath in and four seconds for each breath out.

▣ If you have been practicing lying down, begin to practice in a seated position during the second week.

▣ Once you become comfortable with this type of breathing, try it in a variety of situations (for example, while grocery shopping, watching television, or waiting at red lights).

▣ If you are not sure whether you are still breathing abdominally, put one hand over your upper chest and one just above your navel; the upper hand shouldn't move much, and the lower one should be gently pushed out as you inhale and sink back in as you exhale.

▣ Finally, don't worry too much about doing a perfect job; just be aware of your breathing, and attempt to breathe in a slow and steady way.

Exercise: Logging Your Breathing Retraining

As with all of the skills reviewed in this book, learning to breathe from your abdomen takes practice. To determine whether this is a useful skill for you, make another log in your journal. Record the following: date and time, minutes practiced, anxiety level before each practice, and anxiety level after each practice. For your anxiety ratings, use a scale ranging from 0 (no anxiety) to 100 (as anxious as you can imagine feeling). Here is an example for Gordon.

Date and Time	Minutes Practiced	Anxiety Before Practice	Anxiety After Practice
July 14/8:00 a.m.	10	70	65
July 14/2:00 p.m.	5	55	40
July 14/8:00 p.m.	5	75	40
July 15/8:00 a.m.	10	40	40
July 15/5:00 p.m.	5	55	40
July 15/10:00 p.m.	15	70	25

When Gordon first started learning slow abdominal breathing, he found that it increased his anxiety a bit. This makes perfect sense; we already know that paying attention to our sensations can magnify them. Over the next three months, Gordon found that he was able to practice for longer periods, that these times actually felt calming, and that his general level of day-to-day anxiety seemed to decrease as well.

Progressive Muscle Relaxation

The last strategy discussed in this chapter involves learning to relax the muscles of your body. It was pioneered by Edmund Jacobson in the 1930s (Jacobson 1938) and later refined by Douglas Bernstein and

Thomas Borkovec (Bernstein and Borkovec 1973; Bernstein, Borkovec, and Hazlett-Stevens 2000). This technique, known as *progressive muscle relaxation* (PMR), is useful for a wide range of issues, including stress management, anxiety, insomnia, headaches, anger, and certain types of pain. Jacobson (1938) suggested that a tense mind cannot exist in a relaxed body. The PMR procedures described in this chapter are a variation of those originally developed by Jacobson and by Bernstein and colleagues.

How Does PMR Work?

Initially, PMR involves isolating muscle groups one at a time, purposely tensing the muscles (for about five seconds), and then allowing the area to totally relax (for about twenty to thirty seconds). Tensing the muscle group before releasing the tension provides increased awareness of the tense muscles, helps the person notice the difference between feelings of tension and feelings of relaxation, and provides momentum to enable a deeper state of relaxation. After a fifteen to twenty-five minute session of PMR, many people find themselves much more physically relaxed than they had been before.

Over time, the goal of PMR is for the exercises to become briefer and more portable so that you can use them in situations where you might feel tense or anxious. After a couple of weeks of practicing the full series of relaxation exercises, the next step is to shorten the series to four muscle groups. After that, the next step is to relax these four muscle groups without the tensing exercises. The final stage in the treatment is to relax all of the body's muscles at once.

The initial process. To begin practicing PMR, you can either sit in a comfortable chair or lie down. Loosen any tight clothing, gently close your eyes, and breathe in a slow and relaxed manner (just as you learned in the earlier section on breathing retraining). You will be alternately tensing and relaxing specific groups of muscles. As you relax each muscle group (for twenty to thirty seconds each), try to allow your entire body to become loose and relaxed. Here are instructions for how to tense and relax each major muscle group.

1. *Hands:* Direct your attention to your hands and clench them into tight fists. Hold them for about five seconds, feeling the

tightness. Then suddenly and completely release the muscles, relaxing your hands totally and letting them be limp for twenty to thirty seconds. Straighten and spread your fingers tautly. Hold for five seconds, release, and appreciate the difference in the sensations. Relax.

2. *Arms:* Direct your attention to your arms. To tense your biceps, bend your arms at the elbow, bringing your hands up toward your shoulders and tightening your upper-arm muscles (try not to clench your hands). Hold for five seconds, and then let your arms drop loosely and relaxed to your sides.

3. *Forehead and scalp:* Focus your attention on the top part of your face and head. Raise your eyebrows, wrinkling your forehead. Hold for five seconds and then release, smoothing your forehead. Relax your forehead.

4. *Facial muscles:* Shift your attention down to the muscles of your face: your mouth, and around and under your eyes. Tighten these muscles by scrunching your mouth and closing your eyes. Hold for five seconds (don't forget to breathe), and then release.

5. *Jaw:* Move your attention to the muscles of your jaw. Clench your jaw, feeling the surrounding muscles tense up. Hold for five seconds and then release. Let your mouth fall open, with your jaw loose and relaxed.

6. *Neck and shoulders:* Focus your attention on your neck and shoulders. Pull your shoulders in and up toward your ears. Hold as usual and then release, letting your shoulders droop; feel the tension melt away. Relax. Keep your shoulders in a neutral and relaxed position, and rotate your head slowly to the right until you feel some tension, hold, and then relax. Next rotate to the left, hold, and relax. Tilt your head down and forward, bringing your chin toward your chest until you feel tension. Hold and then relax. Take an extra ten to twenty seconds to mentally run over the muscles you have already

worked on, making sure they are still loose and relaxed. If you notice any areas of tension, release them.

7. *Upper back:* Turn your attention to the area between your shoulder blades, pulling them down and together. Hold for five seconds and then relax.

8. *Stomach:* Gently move your attention to your stomach muscles; tighten them by pulling your stomach in. Again, hold for five seconds and then completely release the muscles. Feel the tension leaving the area as you slowly breathe in and out, in and out.

9. *Buttocks:* Move your attention to your buttocks; tense them, pulling them together. Hold for five seconds and release. Relax and breathe slowly.

10. *Thighs:* Cast your attention onto your thighs. Try not to contract your stomach as you consciously tighten your upper-thigh muscles. Hold for five seconds and release. Feel the tension in your thigh muscles dissipate.

11. *Calves:* Turn your attention to your calf muscles. Point your toes upward, tightening your calves. Hold and release as usual.

12. *Feet:* Finally, focus on your feet. Scrunch your toes together, curling them toward the ground. Hold and release. Feel the tension of your whole body flowing out through your toes, into the floor.

As your PMR practice draws to a close, mentally scan your body for any residual tension. Take a few final moments to unwind completely. Slowly count from one to five, pausing after each number to breathe calmly and to feel your muscles relax more and more completely. After you reach five, you should feel very physically relaxed. For one or two minutes, just remain loose, and breathe slowly and calmly. When you are ready to end your PMR exercise, slowly count backward from five to one, becoming more aware and alert with each number. When you reach two, gently open your eyes. When you reach one, you will be both alert and relaxed.

Exercise: Your PMR Script

To relax and gently work your way through PMR practices, you won't be able to hold this book and read throughout the procedure. So, until you have memorized the script (this usually takes a week or two), there are a few options open to you. You can:

◙ Have a friend or family member read through a PMR script aloud while you practice.

◙ Search online for "progressive muscle relaxation audio" to find a free digital recording that will walk you though the process. Two examples can be found in the resources section at the back of this book.

◙ Check your local bookstore for a PMR tape or CD.

◙ Record your own voice and then play back your script as you practice.

Regardless of your choice, the script will be similar. Next, we have included enough of a script to get you started.

Relax and gently close your eyes. Focus on your breath. Slow and gentle. [Pause.] *In.* [Pause.] *Out. For a moment, just relax and breathe.* [Pause for about a minute.] *Make yourself comfortable. Now, focus your attention on your hands. As you breathe in, clench both hands tightly into fists. Good. Hold it, feel the tension in your fingers, your thumbs, and your wrists.* [Pause.] *Now, let go. Relax your hands. Can you feel the difference? The sudden absence of tension feels pleasant; the tension is draining away. Keeping your hands relaxed, continue to breathe calmly and slowly.* [Pause for twenty to thirty seconds.] *Now flex your hands, spreading your fingers as widely as you can. Good, hold it. Keep holding. Feel the tension in your fingers, across your palm* [pause] *and release.* [Pause for several breaths or about twenty to thirty seconds.]

Continue with this format, tensing each muscle group in the manner just described and then relaxing. Remind yourself (or the other person if you are reading this for a friend) to keep breathing. Although it can be tempting, don't rush through the script; leave plenty of time before progressing to the next muscle group. The whole script should take about twenty minutes. Log your experience (you will find a chart after the next exercise).

PMR Over Time

The goal of PMR is to progress over time from this lengthy and detailed script to feeling able to relax all your muscle groups together—in one step. This is a bit like learning to play the piano: first learning to play melody, then learning chords, and then learning about the pedals; the goal, of course, is to be able to combine these elements. After two weeks of practicing the script as outlined, you may begin to feel that it's becoming easier. You will likely have memorized the process. Once you feel comfortable, it will be time to try combining some of the muscle groups. In doing so, it will take less time and effort to achieve similar results. Weeks three and four will focus on this shorter version of PMR. Instead of tensing each set of muscles separately, work with the following groups:

1. Tense your hands, feet, arms, and legs in the same way as you did during the longer protocol, except that you will tense all of these areas together. Again, hold the tension for about five seconds and then relax these muscles all at once, appreciating the difference between tension and relaxation. Relax for twenty to thirty seconds before moving on to the next groups:

   a. stomach muscles and chest

   b. shoulders

   c. neck, jaw, mouth, and forehead

2. Finally, tense all these muscles together, hold, and release.

You will finish this shortened PMR by again relaxing deeply while counting to five, focusing on your breathing for several minutes, and then becoming increasingly alert as you count backward from five to one.

Log your experience (you will find a chart in the next exercise). After two weeks, you will likely find that this short version has become as effective as the long one was, and you will be ready for the next step, called *relaxation by recall*. For this step, we drop the tension component. Otherwise, the exercise is identical. Instead of tensing each of the four muscle groups, simply focus on the muscle group for five to ten seconds, noticing any tension. Then release any tension you notice, and allow yourself to relax for twenty to thirty seconds before moving on to the next muscle group. Finish the series by deepening your relaxation by counting very slowly from one to five, focusing on your breathing for several minutes, and then becoming increasingly alert as you count back up from five to one. Practice the relaxation-by-recall exercises for about two weeks (weeks five and six).

The final step in PMR is learning to relax all these muscle groups together, as one. This one-step PMR can be useful anywhere and almost anytime. It is fast and simple. Once you are comfortable, take a few slow and calm breaths. After a moment, take notice of any residual tension anywhere in your body, and release it. Feel the tension slide out of your body. For several final moments (if time permits), just focus on your calm and slow breathing. After practicing this one-step PMR in your usual comfortable position, you can start using it in various situations, particularly those in which you experience everyday stresses.

Exercise: Logging Your PMR Practices

Logging will put you in a better position to evaluate whether PMR is right for you. In your journal, make a PMR log like the following example. Most people find that to benefit from this type of relaxation training, they need to practice the technique once or twice a day.

Record the following: date and time, anxiety level before the practice, and anxiety level after the practice. For your anxiety ratings, use a scale ranging from 0 (no anxiety) to 100 (as anxious as you can imagine feeling).

Date and Time	Anxiety Before Practice	Anxiety After Practice
July 14/10:00 a.m.	65	40
July 14/8:00 p.m.	75	40
July 15/10:00 a.m.	50	20
July 15/8:00 p.m.	60	35

Choosing the Techniques That Work Best for You

After you have tried these strategies for a couple of weeks each, spend a few minutes reviewing the three logs you made in this chapter. Based on your subjective sense of which techniques seemed to work best for you, as well as what you recorded in your logs, choose one or two that you are willing to commit to. Carve out a short period each day (or at least a few times a week) to continue your practices. Use your anxiety-management strategy for coping with life's various stresses (like heavy traffic, economic uncertainty, or finding that your partner has left an empty milk carton in the refrigerator—again) and to enhance your overall level of relaxation.

In Brief...

In this chapter you learned the fundamentals of three common and effective anxiety-management strategies; with practice it's quite likely that you will find one that suits you. Dealing with everyday stresses can free up your energy for challenging your health anxiety.

Chapter 7

Medications for Health Anxiety

Although medications are often used to treat anxiety about health, there are virtually no studies of drug treatments for "health anxiety" per se. Rather, research on medication treatments has tended to focus on treating people with particular psychiatric diagnoses, several of which are sometimes associated with health anxiety. For example, people with a diagnosis of *hypochondriasis* are often convinced that they have a serious illness, and may seek reassurance from their doctors, friends, family members, and other sources. People with *panic disorder* are fearful of experiencing rushes of fear or discomfort (panic attacks) out of the blue, and they fear experiencing physical symptoms of arousal, sometimes worrying that these symptoms are a sign that they are about to faint or have a heart attack. People with *generalized anxiety disorder* worry about many areas of their lives, including their work, relationships, money, family, safety, and health, for example. Finally, people with *obsessive-compulsive disorder* sometimes fear becoming ill through contamination from other people or from objects in their environments. There are medications that have been shown to be useful for each of these problems, as well as others. A more detailed discussion of treatments for various anxiety disorders can be found elsewhere (see, for example, *The Anti-Anxiety Workbook*, published by The Guilford Press, 2009).

Before taking medication for health anxiety, it's important to receive a comprehensive diagnostic assessment. Although some medications work for a range of anxiety disorders, others are effective for only certain types of anxiety problems. Therefore, it is possible that any particular medication described in this chapter may not be appropriate for the type of problem you are experiencing. A consultation with a psychiatrist or psychologist is a good first step for establishing an appropriate diagnosis and recommending treatments that are likely to work for your anxiety. Typically, a physician (for example, a family doctor or psychiatrist) is the professional most likely to prescribe medications for anxiety. However, in some jurisdictions, other professionals (such as nurse practitioners) may also treat anxiety-based problems with medication. For the purpose of this chapter, we use the term "doctor" to refer to your prescribing professional, even though this person may not be a physician.

Deciding Whether to Take Medications for Your Anxiety

Research on the treatment of health anxiety and related problems supports psychological approaches (in particular, the cognitive behavioral treatments described in chapters 3 and 4), medication treatments, and combinations of these approaches. In fact, for most anxiety-related problems, cognitive behavioral therapy, medication, and combined treatments are about equally effective, on average (Otto et al. 2009). Of course, for a given person, any one of these approaches may work better than the others. That said, it is difficult to know in advance which treatment is likely to work best for any specific person. One factor that often predicts who will respond best to which treatment is the patient's own expectations and preferences. Your doctor will generally take your preferences into account when recommending one treatment over another.

Cognitive behavioral treatments and medication each have advantages and disadvantages, relative to one another. Medications are easy to take (you just need to swallow a pill), are often less expensive in the short term, and may work more quickly than cognitive and behavioral strategies. On the other hand, CBT tends to have more long-lasting effects than medications; medications are associated with higher relapse rates than CBT, once treatment has ended. As a result, people often take medications longer than they stay in CBT, and medications may be more costly than CBT over the long term. Finally, medications sometimes have unwanted effects on the body that make them difficult for some people to take, including side effects, interactions with other medications, interactions with medical illnesses, and uncomfortable symptoms on discontinuation.

It's not unusual for people with heightened health anxiety to have concerns about taking medication, though these worries are often based more on misconceptions than truth. For example, you may believe that medications for anxiety are dangerous. Although in rare cases medications can trigger serious problems, the medications discussed in this chapter have all been studied extensively to evaluate their effectiveness and safety. When taken as directed by your doctor, these drugs are safe for the majority of people.

Another fear that people have is that the medications will change their personalities or that the side effects will be unbearable. While it's true that some people do experience uncomfortable side effects, most people tolerate the medications described in this chapter very well. In addition, some side effects tend to improve over time. Regardless, side effects are not permanent; they can be eliminated easily by reducing the dosage or discontinuing the medication. Finally, if you fear becoming addicted to medications, it is important to recognize that although some medications for anxiety have the potential for causing physical dependence, most don't. These are issues you can discuss with your doctor and consider in your decisions about whether to try medication and which medications to try.

Strategies for Selecting Medications

A wide range of medications have been found to be effective for reducing anxiety. If you decide to seek medication treatment, your doctor will recommend medications based on a number of different factors. One factor is whether the drug has been found (in placebo-controlled research studies) to be effective for treating the problem you are experiencing. Another is whether the medication is indicated by regulatory bodies, such as the U.S. Food and Drug Administration (FDA), for treating your particular issue. Your doctor will also consider:

- Possible side effects of the drug

- How easy it is to discontinue the drug

- The cost of the medication

- How many times a day the drug needs to be taken

- Whether the medication is likely to interact with other medications you are taking

- Whether the drug is likely to interact with any "recreational drugs" you use (for example, caffeine or alcohol)

- Whether you have a medical condition that might be problematic with a particular drug

- Whether you are planning to become pregnant

Other factors to be considered include your treatment history (for example, which medications you have tried before and whether they were useful) and whether your immediate family members have had a positive response to a particular medication in the past. As you can see, selecting an appropriate medication is a complex process that depends on having a thorough assessment.

Stages of Medication Treatment

There are typically five main stages in medication treatment:

1. Assessment

2. Initiation

3. Acute treatment

4. Maintenance

5. Discontinuation and dose reduction

During the *assessment phase*, your doctor will ask questions to determine the nature of your anxiety problems. Your doctor may also arrange for a physical exam and order a number of tests to rule out possible medical causes for your symptoms. Once you and your doctor have agreed to try medication for your anxiety, the next step is *initiating* the drug. Often, medications are started at low dosages, and the dosage is increased gradually to minimize unwanted side effects. Although lower dosages are often less effective than higher ones, higher dosages are associated with more side effects. Your doctor will try to find a dosage that achieves a balance between maximizing the effectiveness of the drug and minimizing side effects. During the initiation phase, your doctor will monitor your progress to find out whether the drug is having the desired effects. For some medications, it may take several weeks to notice changes in your anxiety.

The *acute treatment phase* refers to the period during which you continue to take the drug at the optimal dosage for the purpose of reducing your anxiety. It is during this phase (typically lasting a few months) that people often see the most improvement. After a person's progress has levelled off, she is likely to continue to take the medication for some time; this period is referred to as the *maintenance phase*. In the case of antidepressants (the most commonly used drugs for anxiety), patients are typically encouraged to continue to take their medications for at least a year, with the assumption that discontinuing the drug too early increases the risk that anxiety symptoms will return.

Many people decide to take their medications for a number of years, and some may never enter into the last phase of medication treatment: the *discontinuation phase*. For most people, the medications discussed in this chapter are believed to be safe for long-term use. However, people often eventually make the decision to discontinue their medications or reduce their dosages. In some cases, this may be because a medication is not working. In other cases, it may be because the person is feeling much better and would prefer to see whether he can now cope with less medication or no medication at all. Some women may also discontinue medication to get pregnant, if there are concerns about the effects of the medication on the developing fetus. Regardless, it's important to discuss the process of discontinuation with your doctor before stopping your medication or changing your dosage. In fact, reducing your medication too abruptly can lead to unpleasant withdrawal effects, and may even be dangerous, depending on the drug. During the discontinuation phase, your doctor will monitor any changes in your anxiety symptoms, as well as any withdrawal symptoms you experience as a result of stopping your medication. For people who have difficulty stopping their medications, cognitive behavioral strategies may help with the process.

Medications for Health Anxiety

Anxiety-based problems, including excessive health anxiety, can be treated using a wide range of medications. Generally, the response to medication treatments varies across people, with some achieving complete relief and others experiencing almost no change. The most typical response to treatment is to experience partial improvement. In other words, most people experience some improvement as a result of treatment but still struggle with anxiety from time to time, even if they continue to take their medications.

The most commonly used drugs for anxiety are antidepressants. Despite their name, antidepressants work for anxiety even if a person is not depressed. In fact, they are used for a wide range of issues other than depression and anxiety, including eating disorders, certain types of pain, and various other problems. The most commonly prescribed antidepressants for anxiety are the *selective serotonin reuptake inhibitors* (SSRIs) and the *serotonin and norepinephrine reuptake inhibitors* (SNRIs). There are other, less commonly used antidepressants as well. Antidepressants usually take four to six weeks to start working.

Another class of drugs that can be used to treat anxiety-based problems is the *benzodiazepines* (a form of antianxiety medication), and there are other types of medication that are sometimes used to treat anxiety as well. In this section, we review commonly used medications for treating problems with health anxiety.

Selective Serotonin Reuptake Inhibitors (SSRIs)

The SSRIs remain one of the most commonly used medications to treat anxiety-based problems. They were first marketed in the early 1980s, with the introduction of fluoxetine. SSRIs that are currently available are listed in the following table, including their generic names, North

American brand names, and suggested dosages (based mostly on recommendations from the Canadian Psychiatric Association) (Swinson et al. 2006).

Generic Name	Brand Name USA/Canada	Suggested Starting Dose	Suggested Maximum Dose
citalopram	Celexa	20 mg	40–60 mg
escitalopram	Lexapro, Cipralex	5–10 mg	20 mg
fluoxetine	Prozac, Sarafem	20 mg	80 mg
fluvoxamine	Luvox	50 mg	300 mg
paroxetine	Paxil	20 mg	60 mg
paroxetine CR	Paxil CR	25 mg	62.5 mg
sertraline	Zoloft	50 mg	200 mg

The SSRIs have been studied extensively for a wide range of anxiety-based problems, including panic disorder, obsessive-compulsive disorder, and generalized anxiety disorder, all of which are sometimes associated with anxiety about health (Swinson et al. 2006). For each of these problems, there is consistent research support for the use of SSRIs, and almost all of the SSRIs are approved by the FDA for treatment of at least one anxiety disorder. Regardless of FDA approval, there is no evidence that any one SSRI is more effective than any other for the treatment of anxiety.

For hypochondriasis, the SSRIs are the only type of drug that has been studied. There have been only two controlled studies of SSRIs for this condition. In one study, fluoxetine was found to be significantly more effective than a *placebo* (an inactive sugar pill) for treating hypochondriasis (Fallon et al. 2008). In another study, CBT and paroxetine were found to be equally effective overall (and superior to placebo) for the treatment of hypochondriasis, though on a few measures, CBT was superior to medication (Greeven et al. 2007). Although these two studies support the use of SSRIs for treating hypochondriasis, there are currently no medications officially approved by the FDA for the treatment of this problem.

SSRIs are believed to work by altering levels of *serotonin* and through their effects on the sensitivity of the serotonin receptors in the brain (serotonin is one of several chemicals in the brain, known as *neurotransmitters*, that transfer information from one nerve cell to the next). The most common side effects of SSRIs include nausea, diarrhea, headache, sweating, anxiety, tremor, sexual dysfunction, weight gain, dry mouth, palpitations, chest pain, dizziness, twitching, constipation, increased appetite, fatigue, thirst, and insomnia. Among people with health anxiety, these symptoms may be mistaken for signs of serious illness. Fortunately, most people experience few of these side effects, and find that the side effects from SSRIs are manageable. Several common SSRI side effects tend to improve within a couple of weeks of starting the medication or increasing the dosage, though other side effects (for example, weight gain and sexual symptoms) tend to continue unless the person decreases the dosage or stops the medication all together.

For the most part, SSRIs can be discontinued with few withdrawal effects. An exception is paroxetine (Paxil), which is processed and eliminated by the body the most quickly relative to other SSRIs. Stopping paroxetine abruptly can lead to uncomfortable flu-like symptoms, so it's important to discontinue the drug gradually. As with any medication, discontinuation of SSRIs should be attempted only with consultation and supervision from your prescribing doctor.

Selective Serotonin and Norepinephrine Reuptake Inhibitors (SNRIs)

There are currently two SNRIs on the market: venlafaxine XR and duloxetine. Brand names for these drugs and suggested dosages (Swinson et al. 2006) are provided in the following table:

Generic Name	Brand Name USA/Canada	Suggested Starting Dose	Suggested Maximum Dose
venlafaxine XR	Effexor XR	37.5–75 mg	225 mg
duloxetine	Cymbalta	20 mg	40–60 mg

Venlafaxine has been found in controlled studies to be effective across a range of health-related anxiety problems, including panic disorder, obsessive-compulsive disorder, and generalized anxiety disorder. Venlafaxine has been approved by the FDA for treatment of several anxiety disorders, though it has not yet been studied in or approved for hypochondriasis. Nevertheless, given the similarity of hypochondriasis to other anxiety-based problems, there is good reason to think this drug might be effective for this condition as well. Duloxetine, a newer SNRI, has been found to be effective for treating generalized anxiety and worry, but has not yet been studied for other anxiety disorders. Generally, the side effects of the SNRIs are similar to those of the SSRIs.

Other Antidepressants

A number of other antidepressants can also be used to treat anxiety disorders. Generally they are not recommended over the SNRIs and SSRIs, either because there is less research supporting them or because the side effects are less favorable (for a review, see Swinson et al. 2006). For example, two older antidepressants, clomipramine (Anafranil) and imipramine (Tofranil) have been found to be useful for treating panic disorder. Clomipramine is also an effective treatment for obsessive-compulsive disorder. However, these drugs are rarely prescribed today, because their side effects are potentially more problematic than those of newer antidepressants, such as the SSRIs and SNRIs. There is also preliminary evidence supporting mirtazapine (Remeron) for some anxiety-based problems, but not enough research to recommend it over the SSRIs and SNRIs for most patients. Finally, bupropion (marketed under the names Wellbutrin and Zyban) is an effective medication for depression, though it doesn't appear to be very helpful for anxiety-based problems.

Benzodiazepines

Considered "minor tranquilizers," benzodiazepines are most frequently prescribed to help people with anxiety problems, insomnia, seizures, alcohol withdrawal, and muscle spasms. Their main effects are to slow down the central nervous system. Although there are more than fifteen benzodiazepines available, only four have been studied extensively for the treatment of anxiety. A list of these medications, including suggested dosages (Swinson et al. 2006), is provided in the following table:

Generic Name	Brand Name USA/Canada	Suggested Starting Dose	Suggested Maximum Dose
alprazolam	Xanax, Niravam	.25 mg	1.5–3 mg
clonazepam	Klonopin, Rivotril	.25 mg	4 mg
diazepam	Valium	2.5 mg	10 mg
lorazepam	Ativan	.5 mg	3–4 mg

Unlike antidepressants (which take a few weeks to have an effect), benzodiazepines begin to work within an hour of taking the drug. They have been shown to help some anxiety disorders (for example, generalized anxiety disorder and panic disorder), but they don't seem to work well for others (such as obsessive-compulsive disorder). Their effects on health anxiety are unknown, but generally they are not recommended as a first option. Rather, SSRI antidepressants are typically recommended first for health anxiety.

A disadvantage of benzodiazepines is that they are often difficult to discontinue. Withdrawal from benzodiazepines often includes anxiety, fear, insomnia, and tremors. Some people also experience seizures when coming off benzodiazepines, particularly if they stop the drug suddenly after long-term use. When stopping a benzodiazepine, it's very important to discontinue the drug gradually and under the supervision of your doctor. This is true of all medications, but especially so for these drugs.

Common side effects of benzodiazepines include sleepiness, lightheadedness, confusion, dizziness, and depression. Some people also experience unsteadiness or memory loss. These drugs should be used with caution in older adults, because they can lead to falling and possibly fractures. Also, these drugs interact strongly with alcohol, so it's important not to combine alcohol with benzodiazepines. Despite the side effects and withdrawal issues associated with benzodiazepine use, many people are able to tolerate taking these drugs for many years without any significant problems. In some cases, combining a benzodiazepine with an SSRI can be useful when first starting a new SSRI. However, once the SSRI kicks in (after four to six weeks), there is often little benefit to taking both drugs, and the benzodiazepine can be discontinued under a doctor's supervision.

Other Antianxiety Medications

There are a number of other medications that are sometimes used to treat anxiety-based problems. For example, buspirone (trade name Buspar) has been found to be useful for generalized anxiety disorder. There is also limited research supporting certain *anticonvulsant* drugs (medications typically used to treat seizures), such as gabapentin (Neurontin) and pregabalin (Lyrica), for particular types of anxiety. At this time, the effects of these drugs on health anxiety are unknown, and they are not recommended as first options for this problem.

Antipsychotic Medications

Antipsychotic medications are used mostly to treat severe mental illness such as schizophrenia. However, in recent years there have been a number of studies suggesting that these drugs can enhance the effects of SSRIs for problems with anxiety and depression. Examples of these drugs (with trade names in parentheses) include risperidone (Risperdal), quetiapine (Seroquel), olanzapine (Zyprexa), ziprasidone (Geodon), and aripiprazole (Abilify). Generally, these are not first-line treatments for anxiety. Rather, they should be reserved for more severe cases of anxiety, or when standard SSRI treatments don't seem to be working on their own. In these cases, combining an SSRI with one of these medications may lead to better outcomes for certain types of anxiety. To date, these drugs have not been studied specifically for health anxiety, however.

Exercise: Keeping a Medication Log

Should you and your doctor decide that a medication trial may be of use in treating your health anxiety, it will be important for you to keep a record of the medications you have tried, dosages, how long you used them, effectiveness, and side effects. This information will be useful in helping your doctor decide whether to:

☑ Continue with a particular medication and dosage.

☑ Increase your dosage.

☑ Decrease your dosage.

☑ Add a medication.

☑ Switch to a different medication.

☑ Discontinue medication treatment altogether.

This information will also be useful if you ever have to see a new doctor or specialist (such as a psychiatrist) in reference to anxiety; appointments are far more useful if you have information about what has and hasn't helped in the past. Finally, information about medication benefits and side effects will come in handy if you find yourself wanting to restart a medication at some point in the future.

At first, it would be best to complete the following medication log daily. After you have been taking a medication with no changes to dosage, effects, or side effects, it may be enough to complete one entry each week or every other week. Regardless, bring this log with you when you return to your prescribing doctor.

Sample Medication Log			
Date	Medication and Dosage	Average Anxiety Level (0 = none, 100 = severe)	Side Effects and Severity (0 = none, 100 = severe)
9/12/11	Citalopram 40 mg	75	Headache (50) Dizziness (10) Fatigue (75)

12/28/11	Citalopram 50 mg	35	Headache (10) Dizziness (10) Fatigue (5)

Herbal Remedies and Alternative Treatments

Increasingly, people are turning to alternative and complementary therapies to deal with various health issues, including anxiety. In fact, a 2002 survey found that 62 percent of adults in the United States had used complementary and alternative remedies in the previous year for a health concern (Barnes et al. 2004). Numerous alternative therapies have been marketed for anxiety, including various herbal remedies, massage, energy therapies, and various other treatments (for a partial list, check out www. holisticonline.com and click on the link for anxiety treatments). However, despite claims that these treatments work, most of these therapies have never been studied systematically. For the few that have been studied, many have been found to be no more effective than placebo.

Nevertheless, there are a small number of herbal supplements (for example, kava, Galphimia glauca, ginkgo biloba special extract Egb 761) that have been found in some studies to be more effective than a placebo for anxiety-based problems. However, evidence has sometimes been mixed (as in the case of kava, for example), or conclusions have been based on very few studies, sometimes of questionable quality (for a review, see Connor and Vaishnavi 2009).

Finally, meditation and aerobic exercise are two alternative treatments that are fairly well supported by research, at least for certain types of anxiety-based issues. To date, however, there are no studies evaluating these approaches to dealing with health anxiety, in particular. In short, much more research is needed before most popular herbal and alternative treatments can be recommended for anxiety problems of any type, let alone health anxiety in particular.

In Brief...

Although several different medications are available for treating anxiety disorders, little research has been conducted on the use of medications for health anxiety in particular. Generally, the first-choice medications for health anxiety are the SSRIs (for example, fluoxetine, paroxetine, escitalopram, sertraline, and so on). The SNRI venlafaxine is also a good option, based on findings with other anxiety-based problems. If these medications don't help or if the side effects are a problem, there are a number of other medication options to choose from. To date, little is known about the effectiveness of most alternative and complementary treatments for anxiety in general, and especially for health anxiety in particular.

Medications may be used on their own or in combination with cognitive and behavioral strategies. For most anxiety problems, CBT, medications, and combinations of these approaches work about equally well in the short term. Over the long term, the effects of CBT appear to be more long lasting than the effects of medication treatments, particularly after treatment has ended.

Resources

Health Anxiety

Asmundson, G. J. G., and S. Taylor. 2005. *It's Not All in Your Head: How Worrying About Your Health Could Be Making You Sick and What You Can Do About It.* New York: The Guilford Press.

Furer, P., J. R. Walker, and M. B. Stein. 2007. *Treating Health Anxiety and Fear of Death: A Practitioner's Guide.* New York: Springer.

Taylor, S., and G. J. G. Asmundson. 2004. *Treating Health Anxiety: A Cognitive-Behavioral Approach.* New York: The Guilford Press.

Willson, R., and D. Veale. 2009. *Overcoming Health Anxiety: A Self-Help Guide Using Cognitive Behavioral Techniques.* London: Constable and Robinson.

Anxiety Self-Help and Cognitive Behavioral Therapy

Antony, M. M., and P. J. Norton. 2009. *The Anti-Anxiety Workbook*. New York: The Guilford Press.

Bourne, E. J. 2011. *Anxiety and Phobia Workbook*. 5th ed. Oakland, CA: New Harbinger Publications.

Burns, D. D. 1999. *The Feeling Good Handbook,* Rev. ed. New York: Plume.

Greenberger, D., and C. Padesky. 1995. *Mind Over Mood: Change How You Feel by Changing the Way You Think*. New York: The Guilford Press.

Mindfulness and Stress Reduction

Davis, M., E. R. Eshelman, and M. McKay. 2008. *The Relaxation and Stress Reduction Workbook*. 6th ed. Oakland, CA: New Harbinger Publications.

Kabat-Zinn, J. 2006. *Mindfulness for Beginners*. CD-ROM. Louisville, CO: Sounds True, Inc.

———. 2009. *Letting Everything Become Your Teacher: 100 Lessons in Mindfulness*. New York: Delta.

Orsillo, S. M., and L. Roemer. 2011. *A Mindful Way Through Anxiety: Break Free from Chronic Worry and Reclaim Your Life*. New York: The Guilford Press.

Progressive Muscle Relaxation Audio Examples

Consortium for Organizational Mental Healthcare. 2010. Positive Coping with Health Conditions: Relaxation Method Audio. www.comh.ca/pchc/resources/audio/index.cfm (accessed February 12, 2011).

Hobart and William Smith Colleges. 2010. Relaxation Techniques: Progressive Relaxation Exercise. http://hws.edu/studentlife/counseling_relax.aspx (accessed February 12, 2011).

References

American College of Emergency Physicians. 2010. *When Should I Go to the Emergency Department?* www.acep.org/practres.aspx?id=26018 (accessed March 14, 2010).

American Psychiatric Association. 2000. *Diagnostic and Statistical Manual of Mental Disorders: DSM-IV-TR.* 4th ed. Text rev. Washington, DC: American Psychiatric Publishing.

Baker, R. C., and D. S. Kirschenbaum. 1993. Self-monitoring may be necessary for successful weight control. *Behavior Therapy* 24 (3):377–94.

Barlow, D. H. 2002. *Anxiety and Its Disorders: The Nature and Treatment of Anxiety and Panic.* 2nd ed. New York: The Guilford Press.

Barnes, P. M., E. Powell-Griner, K. McFann, and R. L. Nahin. 2004. Complementary and alternative medicine use among adults: United States, 2002. *CDC Advance Data Report,* May 27 (343).

Barsky, A. J., and D. K. Ahern. 2004. Cognitive behavior therapy for hypochondriasis: A randomized controlled trial. *Journal of the American Medical Association* 291 (12):1464–70.

Barsky, A. J., E. J. Orav, and D. W. Bates. 2005. Somatization increases medical utilization and costs independent of psychiatric and medical comorbidity. *Archives of General Psychiatry* 62 (8):903–10.

Beck, A. T., and G. Emery. 1985. *Anxiety Disorders and Phobias: A Cognitive Perspective.* With R. L. Greenberg. New York: Basic Books.

Bernstein, D. A., and T. D. Borkovec. 1973. *Progressive Relaxation Training: A Manual for the Helping Professions.* Champaign, IL: Research Press.

Bernstein, D. A., T. D. Borkovec, and H. Hazlett-Stevens. 2000. *New Directions in Progressive Relaxation Training: A Guidebook for Helping Professionals.* Westport, CT: Praeger Publishers.

Connor, K. M., and S. Vaishnavi. 2009. Complementary and alternative approaches to treating anxiety disorders. In *Oxford Handbook of Anxiety and Related Disorders,* ed. M. M. Antony and M. B. Stein, 451–60. New York: Oxford University Press.

Escobar, J. I., L. A. Allen, C. Hoyos Nervi, and M. A. Gara. 2001. General and cross-cultural considerations in a medical setting for patients presenting with medically unexplained symptoms. In *Health Anxiety: Clinical and Research Perspectives on Hypochondriasis and Related Conditions,* ed. G. J. G. Asmundson, S. Taylor, and B. J. Cox, 220–45. Hoboken, NJ: John Wiley and Sons.

Fallon, B. A., E. Petkova, N. Skritskaya, A. Sanchez-Lacay, F. Schneier, D. Vermes, J. Cheng, and M. R. Liebowitz. 2008. A double-masked, placebo-controlled study of fluoxetine for hypochondriasis. *Journal of Clinical Psychopharmacology* 28 (6):638–45.

Furer, P., J. R. Walker, and M. B. Stein. 2007. *Treating Health Anxiety and Fear of Death: A Practitioner's Guide.* New York: Springer.

Greeven, A., A. J. L. M. van Balkom, S. Visser, J. W. Merkelbach, Y. R. van Rood, R. van Dyck, A. J. W. van der Does, F. G. Zitman, and P. Spinhoven. 2007. Cognitive behavior therapy and paroxetine in the treatment of hypochondriasis: A randomized controlled trial. *American Journal of Psychiatry* 164:91–99.

Jacobson, E. 1938. *Progressive Relaxation: A Physiological and Clinical Investigation of Muscular States and Their Significance in Psychology and Medical Practice.* Chicago, IL: University of Chicago Press.

Karoly, P., and W. W. Doyle. 1975. Effects of outcome expectancy and timing of self-monitoring on cigarette smoking. *Journal of Clinical Psychology* 31 (2):351–55.

Locke, E. A. 1968. Toward a theory of task motivation and incentives. *Organizational Behavior and Human Performance* 3:157–89.

Miller, W. R., and S. Rollnick. 2002. *Motivational Interviewing: Preparing People for Change.* 2nd ed. New York: The Guilford Press.

Moscovitch, D. A., M. M. Antony, and R. P. Swinson. 2009. Exposure-based treatments for anxiety disorders: Theory and process. In *Oxford Handbook of Anxiety and Related Disorders,* ed. M. M. Antony and M. B. Stein, 461–75. New York: Oxford University Press.

Orsillo, S. M., and L. Roemer. 2011. *The Mindful Way Through Anxiety: Break Free from Chronic Worry and Reclaim Your Life.* New York: The Guilford Press.

Otto, M. W., E. Behar, J. A. J. Smits, and S. G. Hofmann. 2009. Combining pharmacological and cognitive behavioral therapy in the treatment of anxiety disorders. In *Oxford Handbook of Anxiety and Related Disorders,* ed. M. M. Antony and M. B. Stein, 429–40. New York: Oxford University Press.

Prochaska, J. O., and C. C. DiClemente. 1983. Stages and processes of self-change of smoking: Toward an integrative model of change. *Journal of Consulting and Clinical Psychology* 51 (3):390–95.

Salkovskis, P. M., H. M. C. Warwick, and A. C. Deale. 2003. Cognitive-behavioral treatment for severe and persistent health anxiety (hypo-chondriasis). *Brief Treatment and Crisis Intervention* 3:353–68.

Sturmey, P., and M. Hersen, eds. In press. *Handbook of Evidence-Based Practice in Clinical Psychology: Volume II—Adult Disorders.* Hoboken, NJ: John Wiley and Sons.

Swinson, R. P., M. M. Antony, P. Bleau, P. Chokka, M. Craven, A. Fallu, M. Katzman, K. Kjernisted, R. Lanius, K. Manassis, D. McIntosh, J. Plamondon, K. Rabheru, M. van Ameringen, and J. R. Walker. 2006. Clinical practice guidelines: Management of anxiety disorders. *Canadian Journal of Psychiatry* 51 (Suppl. 2):1S–92S.

Taylor, S., and G. J. G. Asmundson. 2004. *Treating Health Anxiety: A Cognitive-Behavioral Approach.* New York: The Guilford Press.

Taylor, S., D. S. Thordarson, K. L. Jang, and G. J. G. Asmundson. 2006. Genetic and environmental origins of health anxiety: A twin study. *World Psychiatry* 5 (1):47–50.

U.S. Department of Health and Human Services. 1999. *Mental Health: A Report of the Surgeon General.* Rockville, MD: U.S. Department of Health and Human Services, Substance Abuse and Mental Health Services Administration, Center for Mental Health Services, National Institutes of Health, National Institute of Mental Health.

Walker, J. R., N. Vincent, and P. Furer. 2009. Self-help treatments for anxiety disorders. In *Oxford Handbook of Anxiety and Related disorders*, ed. M. M. Antony and M. B. Stein, 488–96. New York: Oxford University Press.

Williams, M., J. Teasdale, Z. Segal, and J. Kabat-Zinn. 2007. *The Mindful Way Through Depression: Freeing Yourself from Chronic Unhappiness.* New York: The Guilford Press.

Katherine M. B. Owens, PhD, is adjunct professor at the University of Regina and clinical lecturer at the University of Saskatchewan. Clinically, Owens serves as a senior psychologist in the Regina Qu'Appelle Health Region Mental Health Clinic and as a therapist in private practice. She practices, teaches, and supervises psychology and psychiatry students in the cognitive behavioral model, specializing in anxiety disorders, depression, and neuropsychological assessment. In her spare time, Owens volunteers as much as she can.

Martin M. Antony, PhD, is professor and director of graduate training at Ryerson University in Toronto, Canada. He is also director of research at the Anxiety Treatment and Research Centre at St. Joseph's Healthcare, Hamilton, Ontario, and Past President of the Canadian Psychological Association. An award-winning researcher, Antony is coauthor of *The Anti-Anxiety Workbook, When Perfect Isn't Good Enough,* and more than twenty-five other books. His research, writing, and clinical practice focus on cognitive behavioral therapy and the treatment of anxiety disorders. He has been widely quoted in the American and Canadian media.

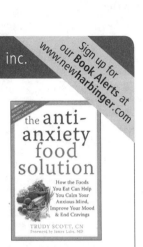
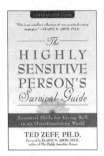

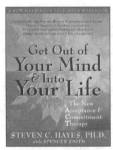
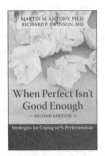
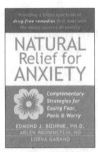